PAIN CONTROL

The Bethesda Program

PAIN CONTROL
The Bethesda Program

Bruce Smoller, M.D.
and Brian Schulman, M.D.

Doubleday & Company, Inc.
Garden City, New York   1982

To the Smollers—Cozy, Jamie, and Lauren—and the
Schulmans—Cookie, Beth, and Lisa—who motivated
our efforts, encouraged our progress, waited patiently
through months of work away from home, and always
believed in our project

Library of Congress Cataloging in Publication Data

Smoller, Bruce.
Pain control: the Bethesda program.

Bibliography: p. 289
Includes index.
1. Pain—Prevention.   2. Pain—Psychological aspects.
I. Schulman, Brian.   II. Title.
RB127.S63   616'.0472
AACR2
ISBN: 0-385-17252-4
Library of Congress Catalog Card Number 81–43299

Drawings by Lisa Larson

ACKNOWLEDGMENTS

The preparation of this book about people required untold hours of assistance, encouragement, and research by some very special people. We would like to extend our thanks and appreciation to them. For technical assistance and help in organizing the volumes of technical data, our thanks go to Dr. Richard Gracely, Dr. Steven Targum, Dr. Barry Jay Kirshner, and to the members of the Pain Study Program at the National Institute of Dental Research of the National Institutes of Health. Special thanks to Dr. Arnold Binderman for his contributions to the section on temporomandibular joint dysfunction.

For the preparation of the manuscript, we thank Susan Bell, our chief organizer, and also Francis Miller, Barbara Levine, Joyce Richardson, Lucille Perodeau, Marilyn Mehr, Jane Thomas, Michelle Kelley, and the staff of the Raytheon Service Company. Our thanks go to Lisa Larson for her magnificent illustrations, to Nan Grubbs, our editor at Doubleday, for her valuable assistance and support, and to Anita Diamant, who helped make the book a reality.

Special thanks to Cookie Schulman and Cozy Smoller, who, as wives and as health care professionals, were able to editorially comment on and assess our work; to the hundreds of patients under our care who helped contribute to our knowledge and understanding of the human dimension of pain problems; and finally to Ruth Hume, who pointed us in the right direction and whose grace in the face of severe pain was inspirational.

BRUCE SMOLLER
BRIAN SCHULMAN

CONTENTS

III   GETTING OFF THE PAIN-GO-ROUND:
      CREATING A PERSONAL PAIN
      CONTROL PROGRAM

Appendices

INTRODUCTION

Think of all the things that are important to you: loved ones, a career, a family, sports, exercise, friends, maintaining a home, a satisfactory sex life, a sense of humor, a good night's sleep, a sense of worth. Write these down on a piece of paper. Now you could order these things in terms of importance, setting priorities, and deciding what is most important. If you have chronic pain, however, you don't have to worry about ordering the list; you can just crumple it and throw it away. Order is not important, because chronic pain robs you of all these things. If your pain was once an unpleasant sensation, now it is much more. It is the shrunken remnant of what you valued in life. Chronic pain divides the world in two: the "haves," those who live in pain, and the "have nots," who are blessed to be free from pain. For those who have pain, suffering is very real, and part of daily life. The "have nots" do not bear such a burden and they assume that with time and good medical care, the "haves' " pain will simply go away.

The medical miracles we constantly hear about increase our confidence in doctors' know-how to fix us when we break. Although we accept that the doctors are still working on major breakdowns like cancer, we assume that they have no trouble with everyday repairs like a strained back or an inflamed joint. No one has to tell you how this fairy tale is totally shattered when pain strikes. Suddenly you find that medicine does not have the answer to everything, and that the answers you do get are not even the same from doctor to doctor. You are trapped in a cave, screaming to get out, but no one hears you. The "have nots" do not understand. They mean well when they ask, "How are you doing?" But how do you answer? With the truth or a happy face? No wonder it is often easier to avoid the "have nots," those people who used to be your friends, acquaintances, and coworkers. But the innocent "How are you doing?" is nothing compared to the message that medicine often gives you: "I can't find the cause. I can't find the cure. Maybe it is in your head." How outrageous! You suffer with pain, yet you have to prove it to others. It is as if you are guilty until proved innocent. Sometimes you envy the handicapped. At least they do not have to *prove* their problems, doctors and friends do not doubt their word.

All of us, both the "haves" and the "have nots," like to view life in simple terms. We all like things neat and easy. We all want something we can see, define. This tendency to view the world in simple, physical terms is why we think of, or once thought of, our bodies as a car that the doctor-mechanic just fixes. It is why we would envy the handicapped: the existence of their problem is clear, simple, and visible to all. That is why physical signs of pain (a brace, a surgical scar, the need to take medication) are so appealing. The "have nots" can never see *your* real problem. It is the invisibility of your pain, and your uncertainty about the length of its duration, that sets you apart from others.

Pain Control was not written for doctors or scientists, but for you, the "haves" of chronic pain. It provides a sound and practical plan for the management of chronic pain.

Successful treatment of chronic pain involves much more than alleviating distressing sensations. It includes attention to those facets of life fractured by the struggle with pain. Unfortunately doctors, pills, and surgical procedures alone cannot restore these important parts of life. *You* are needed to repair this type of damage. Reaching this understanding is a major step toward management of your pain problem.

RICHARD H. GRACELY, PH.D.
Research Psychologist,
National Institutes of Health;
clinical pain specialist
in private practice

PAIN: AN OVERVIEW

This is a book on how to treat pain. Pain which is chronic, persistent, and nagging. Pain which does not respond to aspirin or other pain-killers, which ignores heat, defies massage, depresses your mood, shortens tempers, allows your kids to irritate you, ruins your sex life, and saps your spouse's last ounce of patience. It is the type of pain that leads you to every medical specialist in town, perhaps even some out of town; through an assortment of X rays, myelograms, scans, and blood tests; makes you consider surgery, acupuncture, and hypnosis, and, at moments, even consider giving up.

At times it is clearly worse, occasionally it is better, but it never goes away. It persists—an uninvited guest—rampaging through your body.

Perhaps on one occasion a physician suggested that it was a disk problem, but the myelogram showed nothing. Another doctor diagnosed arthritis. A specialist said it was arachnoiditis with some bursitis. Each attack caused an inflammation, a temporary exacerbation, a journey from bad to worse. Most of the time, no one knows what to do for you. When someone has a suggestion, it just does not work. Doctors have assured you it is not cancer, but no one seems to know what it is or how to relieve it.

You are caught in an endless cycle of pain. It accompanies you to bed, distresses your sleep, and awakens you in the morning. Such is chronic, benign, intractable pain. It may start as a backache, a headache, or a stiff neck, but eventually it progresses, adversely affecting your physical health and emotional well-being. It does not let up; it gets all of you.

THE CUTTING EDGE OF PAIN

Pain is the screaming of our body to our mind. It is a loud and unsettling call. Pain hurts. It will not be ignored. As an internal communication, it is first and foremost a symptom—the body's alarm system. As a symptom, it is the most common complaint that brings a patient to a doctor. Examining and analyzing pain may provide the physician valuable clues in his medical examination. The intensity, duration, radiation, and frequency of pain are all potentially important parameters for studying the extent and progress of disease processes. Acute pain is the most urgent of our body's warnings, signaling danger, forcing ameliorative action.

Acute pain may be persistent pain. Such pain may be the tenacious, debilitating companion of progressive, malignant disease. As cancer spreads, encroaching on the territorial integrity of normal tissue structure, severe pain may occur. For the cancer patient with intractable pain, hope resides in the generous and appropriate use of potent narcotic analgesics as well as the potential resources of neurosurgical ablation (the surgical destruction of central pain centers). Such humanitarian and scientifically valid treatment is indicated and should be readily employed in the management of intractable pain.

But not all pain is acute, a warning of tissue injury. Nor is all pain intractable, the concomitant of malignant disease. Far and away the most common pain problems involve chronic, benign pain. This pain may originate from a genuine physical source (arthritis, neuritis, weakness of the back, etc.) or may have started as the symptom of a disease, but in a subtle and progressive manner it began to outshout the disease. Like an alarm bell stuck in the "on" position it persists, continuing to signal danger long after the cessation of genuine threat. Such is chronic benign pain: it is a continuous, repetitive message of discomfort that, over time, exceeds its function as a symptom of disease and injury. Chronic pain *becomes* the disease and in its wake brings a new and potentially devastating array of health problems.

In considering pain management one must always bear in mind the origin of pain. But pain cannot be completely or comprehensibly understood solely on the basis of its origin. Pain exists as a process —a regulatory force influencing the course and conduct of an individual's life. Even for the cancer patient, where the progression of disease is constantly creating new pain, it is limiting to automatically ascribe the total pain experience to the malignancy. Chronic pain processes may coexist, contributing to the individual's distress.

The cutting edge of pain is the razorlike effect of pain as it shears away at the emotional stability and social structure of a person. Experiencing the immediate distress of actually hurting is, in itself, distressing. But *living* in pain, contending with the responsibilities of day-to-day life under the constant stress of pain, creates the real destructive potential of chronic pain. Stress-induced illness, mental illness, loss of the ability to work, even substance abuse, are but some of the most common complications of chronic pain. Their aftermath can affect every aspect of a person's life.

REAL PEOPLE, REAL PAIN

Alvin Busch is forty-two years old. For sixteen years he was the regional manager of a merchandising business in Washington, D.C. For six of those sixteen years, he received a meritorious service award and a substantial bonus for his services. He was highly regarded as an industrious, creative manager, someone uniquely qualified to handle stress. Alvin was in excellent physical condition. An avid tennis player, he had won the B division title at his country club on two occasions in the past five years. Winter vacations were spent skiing in Colorado with his wife and two teenage sons.

Last week, Alvin Busch, under fire, resigned. For the past nine months he has been unable to work because of back spasms and headaches. For the first forty-one and one half years of his life, he never missed a day of school or called into work sick because of ill health. For Alvin, pain was something he felt for a moment after stubbing a toe. Aspirin was used on occasion to chase a lingering hangover. Simply, until now, Alvin Busch has never been sick. He resigned because the residual effects of a fall on a newly waxed floor left him with pain radiating down the back of both legs—making sitting a torment, driving the car for any distance a risk, and physical activity of any duration virtually exhausting. Although mentally fit, he could no longer keep up with the physical strain of his position. Despite regular physical therapy, antispasmodics, and analgesics, the pain and its constant aggravation did not significantly change.

After sixteen years on the job, Alvin Busch woke up one morning unable to dress himself, shave and shower, and get to work without significant pain and discomfort. What had begun as a minor fall nine months previously had become a major life tragedy. For Alvin Busch, and 40 million Americans with chronic pain, the real toll of pain is not in the billions of dollars spent seeking relief, but in the time lost from productive work, the absence of physical activities and pleasurable recreation, and the constant mental and physical strain of persistent discomfort.

We knew Alvin Busch. He was not a coward; his courage and fortitude were often exceptional. He made the most of his job by putting himself into everything he did. Always willing to give 100 percent, he did not hold back. Alvin could not conceive of slowing down or in any way altering the physical aspects of his job. The toughness suited him; he was an athlete, a man who did everything to win. He pulled no punches. Changing pace, slowing down to accommodate himself to his pain problem, was not his style. His personality was set in cement.

Al went to college in the early fifties. He lived through the basketball scandals. His life centered around college basketball. He loved sports. The night Ralph Beard, a famous college basketball player of the fifties, admitted taking five hundred bucks as a bribe to shave points, Al Busch cried. He thought it was the worst thing that had ever happened in his whole life. The man he thought was the most superb guard who ever played the game was a fake. The revelation broke his heart and he made up his bull-headed mind to dedicate himself totally to his own career. The scandals shaped his life; he would never shave points.

When he got hurt and found the physical aspects of his work too demanding, he considered the season over. "Doc, what am I going to do? If I can't go back and do the job they pay me for, then I won't work." Once again, Al Busch had made up his mind.

In March 1978, he retired to Florida. To the best of our knowledge, he hasn't worked since.

THE EPIDEMIC OF CHRONIC PAIN

Alvin Busch is no different from a lot of other people we have come to know in our work. He was a normal, healthy guy with a good job, more than a bit of ambition, and the desire to make something out of his life. For Alvin, the injury that precipitated his pain was trivial—an acrobatic tumble across a newly waxed floor. Only the consequence was major: an early retirement to Florida and a lifetime of chronic pain.

Many people are quite familiar with chronic pain. It is the third leading cause of disability in the United States, ranking just below cancer and heart disease. But pain is probably the least understood major health problem. Until very recently, little research money was devoted to trying to understand the unique problems and complications of chronic pain. The tide, however, is turning, and, in 1980 the directors of the prestigious Association for Research in Nervous and Mental Diseases felt strongly enough about the importance of pain research to declare pain "the most pressing human health problem facing Americans in the 1980s" and devoted their entire fifty-eighth annual meeting to vital areas of pain research.

As unpleasant as it may be to contemplate, you or someone in your family will probably have a chronic pain problem. At present, there are 40 million Americans who suffer from the various sequelae of chronic pain. Historically, very little emphasis was placed on prevention; the focus of attention and money was given to the medical care and compensation of pain victims who were disabled and in need of treatment. Pain as a burden is enormous. The cost of compensating pain sufferers in 1981 was estimated to be $20 billion. Including the loss of productivity, the annual cost rises to a staggering $50 billion. That is a huge expense—but it does not even begin to measure the extent of human suffering and conflict.

Pain compensation is a national disaster. Just consider the following:

▪ Five million people are disabled by *low back pain*. They will pay $1.5 billion in hospital and doctor bills, which includes 200,000 surgical procedures and nearly 19 million visits to doctors.
▪ The average American loses two weeks of productivity per year due to pain.
▪ Over $1 billion in over-the-counter pain medications are sold each year.
▪ Each year $400 million in the habit-forming, enormously addictive drug codeine proporythene are sold.

These statistics are staggering. Can anything really be done or must pain casualties be tolerated as an unavoidable consequence of disease and injury? Despite the phenomenal development of sophisticated medical technology, there are many people who have suffered for years without substantial relief. The longer pain persists, the more tenacious and debilitating it becomes. Pain is a virulent predator: it rapidly pursues, engulfs, and incapacitates its victims.

Alvin Busch was an unwilling victim: in a way, the perfect foil. A healthy young man with a bright future, he got caught on the pain-go-round, found no relief, and decided, with considerable reluctance, to retire. His loss is a national tragedy. He had plenty left to contribute but could not change views and redirect his energies. Pain can freeze a personality in much the same way it freezes a joint. People in pain get stuck and begin to chase hopes and promises, eventually finding only disappointment, frustration, and more pain. It is the chase, the quest for pain eradication, that leads one to hopelessness and disability.

If anything, Alvin was too determined. The record reads that he retired due to "chronic pain secondary to lumbosacral strain." The reality is that society lost one productive, competent worker because he got hurt and could not change gears. Certainly he had pain, but it was not pain that disabled him: it was the same hard-nosed, stubborn work ethic that propelled him to a position of managerial responsibility that ultimately did him in. Such is the irony of chronic pain.

CHRONIC PAIN: A SPECIAL PROBLEM

One major problem is that pain is not a disease like pneumonia, hypertension, or gastritis, where it is often easy to isolate the offending pathogens and implement an appropriate course of therapy. Pain is a syndrome, a group of related symptoms. There is no clinical test to verify its presence or measure its intensity. The patient can only tell the doctor what he feels and hope, often futilely, that the doctor can help him control the feeling. While doctors are often very able diagnosticians of diseases that they know about, they are not mind readers and cannot recommend treatment for something they simply cannot see, feel, measure, or completely understand.

Several years ago, while watching a television documentary ceremoniously belaboring the arduous course of medical students, we were struck with an immediate sense of recognition. In one respect, it was consoling to see that tradition lived on and that others were enduring similar image-shattering tribulations. We watched the students scurry through emergency rooms, across hospital wards late at night, attending to the manifold difficulties of critically ill people. The familiarity of person, place, and circumstance was reassuring. But beneath that veil of urgency, emergency, and crisis, we had a primal inkling that there were characters other than the students in this drama. There they were, lying on stretchers, sitting on beds, sitting about halls on overstuffed chairs. They had suffered heart attacks, gunshot wounds; they were there being resuscitated or awaiting intubation, tests, X rays, and the like. While not at the center of this drama, they were certainly the focus of the student-protagonists' attempted craftsmanship. While all emotional resonance was focused on the students, the central characters were actually the patients. At the center of this tale of young scientists learning to be doctors were real live people who happened to be sick.

When one is very busy being a doctor, it is easy to forget and at times almost impossible to allow oneself to see that at the other end of doctoring is a real person: a being with feelings, needs, and fears. That person is someone with a family who loves him and cares very much about what happens to him. Sometimes doctors forget that patients are people.

Only grudgingly do we share this insight. In a way, it is embarrassing; medicine is, after all, the healing art, the giving from one person to another. It is not easy to admit that the "other" part of that relationship is not always well considered.

Generally, however, doctors cannot be accused of inattention to pain problems. They consider patients' complaints quite seriously and vigorously pursue the diagnosis and treatment of even the most seemingly benign pain complaint. Nonetheless, the temptation to provide relief can often exceed the professional's capabilities. Frequently, the sympathetic doctor confronted with the anguished patient may promise to do more than he is reasonably able to do.

When we are ill and seek help from the doctor, we desire not only relief but also reassurance. As dependent creatures, a finite amount of certainty is required to feel comfortable. We want to know why we hurt, what will make it better, and how long the process will take. Confidence in a doctor and his ability to accurately predict the course of events often go hand in hand.

For the most part, controlling chronic pain is enigmatic. Despite the enormous advances in medical technology, and the sophisticated diagnostic tests, it is often impossible to determine why pain varies from day to day or persists in spite of apparently adequate treatment. This makes patients unhappy. The absence of a physical diagnosis creates anxiety which increases the pain. With anxiety comes the demand for certainty and invariably a call for more tests. Consequently, when a patient is evaluated for pain problems he may feel an initial skepticism for any diagnosis and subsequent treatment that does not specifically focus on a part of the anatomy. The most popular therapies are those that distinguish, isolate, and eventually eliminate a physical source of discomfort. In general, we are pleased knowing that whatever is wrong might be aided by bandaging, massaging, splinting, or removing a peripheral and nonessential part of the anatomy.

The idea that pain and pain alone can be a disease is relatively new and not particularly well accepted by the vast majority of people. We are not only fearful of pain, but are shameful of having pain without also having a "real"—i.e., physical—cause for that pain.

Consequently, physicians find themselves under considerable pressure to identify the physical cause of a patient's pain. Fortunately for the belabored and besieged physicians, many people with chronic pain often do have a physical disease or injury, such as arthritis, degenerative joint or disk disease, vascular headaches, or any one of the degenerative processes of normal aging. Hence, the diagnostic search for underlying physical problems is often fruitful. But the doctor may diagnose an illness, recommend therapy, perhaps prescribe a medication or two, and still the pain persists. In some cases treating the underlying condition may even make the pain worse. Often, despite the very best of available treatments, chronic pain problems persist, anguishing the patient and frustrating the doctor.

The bottom line is that no single treatment seems to help. The patient with pain rapidly becomes the person with chronic pain going from specialist to specialist, constantly seeking new medication, better, more effective physical treatments, and the ultimate eradication of the pain. This marks the start of the endless cycle of pain, promise, and disappointment.

SEARCHING FOR HELP

For many, pain is a lonely experience. Living in constant pain is a dreadful state of affairs. Not wanting to be with people lest they sense your discomfort, or to go anywhere for fear of becoming even more aware of your own discomfort, leads to a restriction of activities and a monochromatic and distorted perspective. Life quickly becomes dull and boring. Coping ability is impaired as excessive introspection and self-absorption blur the boundaries of reality and distort good judgment.

Fantasy and the fearful creations of intense imagination can easily absorb the person living in pain. The tendency toward isolation is extreme. Sitting at home day after day, stuck outside the productive mainstream, the pain patient may feel alone and at times abandoned. Guilt, anxiety, and shame—the products of helplessness—become constant companions. Often the person in pain wishes for something tangible to demonstrate his distress. Under stress, he doubts himself and questions his credibility, finding it difficult to understand his own dilemma: "How can pain persist? Why do I suffer despite all I do?" He wonders how anyone else could ever believe him. Doubt clouds judgment, fear erodes confidence, and living with people becomes a burden. The person living in pain may feel defenseless and accused. Facing an endless stream of well-wishers, benevolent friends trying to be helpful, who ask "What is wrong with your neck?" "Are you feeling any better this week?" "When do you think you'll be going back to work?" only intensifies the conflict.

A young woman suffering with the residual pain of a whiplash injury described the course of personal retreat rather succinctly:

After a while it becomes a chore to remain polite. My patience grew thin. I began to lose my composure. My temper would flare just over ordinary little things. It became easier to simply withdraw; not only from friends, but family as well. I discovered my bedroom had a door that shuts and locks. Retreating to my bedroom became the answer to a host of unpleasant, unsolicited intrusions. Not being at dinner beats having to explain feeling poorly. I would do anything to avoid confrontations. After all, no one could understand, not even my husband.

Ten minutes before he arrived home from work I would go upstairs and pretend to be asleep. I was frightened that he would ask me how I felt. Something simple like that just terrified me. I spent hours thinking about it. I wanted to smack him. I knew he didn't believe me. How could he? After all, I didn't believe it myself. He was always so sweet. I knew it was false, he didn't want to upset me, tell me to get off my behind and do something constructive. At times I felt he was treating me like a child. At times I felt like a child.

Turning the Tide: Chronic Pain Reconsidered

Over the past ten years, a new emphasis has been placed on pain as a protean health problem. In medical terms, we now conceive of chronic pain as a multisystem disorder, one affecting a number of physical and emotional functions. The term *chronic benign pain syndrome* has gained popularity as descriptive of this composite process.

A major breakthrough in pain treatment has resulted from the collaborative efforts of allied medical specialists who are now approaching chronic pain as a multisystem process. Recognizing the physical origins of pain as the nidus but not the totality of the disease process, pain treatment teams employ a comprehensive treatment approach to pain management. Operating primarily out of large, university-affiliated medical centers, organized primarily as time-limited inpatient programs, these programs have enabled many pain sufferers to receive expert consultation and have, for many, initiated meaningful treatment programs. The goals of these programs are generally threefold: to identify and eliminate positive reinforcers of pain behavior, to increase physical activity, and to decrease excessive drug use.

This multispecialty pain approach has received considerable media attention and has helped to increase public awareness of newer pain therapies as well as to facilitate the medical community's gradual acceptance of a multidisciplinary approach to pain management. The spawning and dissemination of the pain clinic concept suggests acceptance of specific pain therapies aimed at treating the human consequences of pain. The growth of pain clinics has been phenomenal. In 1970, there were only two clinics in operation in the United States; by 1980, there were over three hundred. Virtually every major hospital and medical center now has plans for establishing a definitive pain treatment program. The reason, quite simply, is the growth of public demand. Chronic pain is beginning to achieve recognition as a major health problem. It is finally being recognized as a disease.

THE BETHESDA PROGRAM

As a function of our collective backgrounds including training in medicine, orthopedics, and psychiatry, we find ourselves at a unique focal point along the mind-body continuum. As physicians, we understand the anatomical structure and physiological functioning of the human body. We have eagerly followed the scientific developments that have revolutionized medical knowledge over the past twenty years, and have tried to incorporate genuine biologic discoveries into our clinical practice. Yet, as psychiatrists, we are also specifically concerned with the psychological factors that influence health and disease.

As we have gained experience working with people who were referred to us specifically for pain control, we have become distinctly aware of the diverse consequences of living in pain. Every person requires a thorough history and a review of medical records. Each receives an extensive physical and psychological examination (as well as a family interview), a complete physical and neurological examination, and whatever laboratory tests are indicated. Understanding people the way we feel they need to be understood isn't easy: it takes a great deal of time and effort. In the process we have learned a great deal about chronic pain and how it affects people's health. In the end, we have come to appreciate the uniqueness of each patient and to truly respect the differences between people.

The guiding principle of our program resides in the belief that the patient's role in his own treatment is central to the overall health care effort. The patient must assume responsibility for the control of his pain. The delegation of primary responsibility to the physician creates excessive dependency and can initiate a passive behavior pattern leading to unwarranted and unsuccessful treatments. In this regard, the pain patient must understand the nature of his pain and how various treatments may potentially offer pain control. The first section of our book offers the reader a simple but comprehensive overview of the mechanisms of pain. We do not expect our readers to be physicians or experts, but simply to be informed. There are far too many misconceptions and distortions that surround the pain syndrome. A little clarification can go a long way in helping to control pain.

The second principle of treatment encompasses understanding pain as a uniquely human event. Living in pain is punishing and creates a multitude of health problems. Psychiatry has long appreciated the importance of human emotions in regulating behavior and well-being. The second section of this book explains how living in pain can shear the fabric of a person's life and erode his sense of well-being. Successful pain control requires an understanding of the natural history of persistent pain and what specific steps must be taken to halt the progression of its cutting edge.

The third principle of treatment regards pain as a multisystem disorder affecting physical and psychological processes. We share the view that much pain is a learned maladaptive behavior which is reinforced by conditioned responses, ineffectual therapies, poor physical condition, the abuse and misuse of medication, emotional stress, anxiety, and poor nutrition. In Section 3, we provide a step-by-step breakdown of the various pain reinforcers and enhancers that commonly trouble patients, and a practical framework for creating an individual pain program and a meaningful record of personal pain progress. This program can be used as an adjunct to whatever therapy your personal physician may institute.

We strongly believe that the successful completion of the personal record may be the single most important factor in aiding the patient to deal with his pain problems. The diary will become a personal source for pain information, detailing accurate data regarding medication benefits and drawbacks, pain enhancers and reducers, actual pain experiences, and much more. Upon completion of the diary, you can show your physician an exact medical record of the pain problem and documentation of the effects of the various therapies. The diary is an accurate clinical record and a meaningful basis for recommending appropriate treatment.

A FINAL NOTE

We have far too much respect for the tenacity of chronic pain to promise any simplistic, homespun remedies.

The more we learn about the complexity of chronic illness and the enormous potential that it harbors for partial and permanent disability, the more vital the demand for a "participant" effort becomes. To survive, you must progress. Standing still, not improving, will produce regressive changes. It is no longer adequate to visit a physician, describe your various aches and pains, and then, without any effort on your part, expect relief. Chronic pain conditions are far too complex to allow simple, effortless solutions.

We have come to believe that time is the most important element in the fight to control chronic pain. As time passes and a person with pain remains bedridden, homebound, or simply out of work, the likelihood of ever getting well rapidly dwindles.

Although we may seek solace in the adage that time heals all wounds, much depends on how our time is spent. Idleness and procrastination waste time, stealing away the most precious of human gifts. For time to heal, it must work to create a positive experience. A person with pain is in a race against time. The words of Franklin Delano Roosevelt "Never before have we had so little time in which to do so much" aptly apply to the battle against pain.

Yet people walk around in pain, shopping from doctor to doctor seeking new medications, better diagnoses, anything informative upon which to hang a hope or two. People walk around as if there were years to waste beating the bushes, with a single goal in mind: trying to find the key to a pain-free life.

A personal strategy is a prerequisite to healing. Belief in the positive value of human emotions is essential. You cannot get well unless you believe you have control over the process. For years, medical researchers have studied and scientifically documented the effects of excessive stress in the development of illness. Hypertension, heart disease, peptic ulcers, even cancer, are all potential end products of chronic exposure to excessive, unmitigated stress. Now, finally, we are beginning to more fully appreciate the potential for coping and adaptation as creative mechanisms in managing pain. The discovery of the body's own natural pain-killers is but the initial step in unraveling the mind-body mystery.

Good health begins in the mind. The messages we send our body regulate every conscious, unconscious, and involuntary action of our body. Do not underestimate the importance of the mind in the battle to conquer pain. It is the master control and its potential is limitless.

Getting off the pain-go-round is your choice. We hope that the Bethesda Pain Control Program will provide an avenue by which you can begin to control the problems that have controlled you for so long. If you desire to participate it will not be easy, but now as always, the choice is yours.

I

FROM ACHES TO PAINS: GETTING CAUGHT ON THE PAIN-GO-ROUND

Chapter 1

SEVEN QUESTIONS

The following questions are the most frequently asked in our practice. At first sight, answering them can be deceptively simple. On reflection, however, they contain a distillation of the fears, needs, and expectations common to people in pain. Sometimes a response poses more questions than it answers. Exploring some of these issues should prove useful.

QUESTION NO. 1

Is My Pain Real?

The Most Commonly Asked Question

Because pain cannot, as yet, be directly measured, persons affected by chronic pain often begin to wonder if their pain is real. Sometimes that feeling is magnified by well-meaning friends, family, and even doctors. For many years, the medical community approached chronic pain problems as if they were either a physical or an emotional problem—not both. Pain complaints have been labeled either "genuine," originating from a real pain source (arthritic joint, slipped or ruptured disk, etc.), or "functional"—connoting the function of a healthy imagination. We live under the illusion of a mind-body division. Dividing mind from body, however, results in a fruitless quest for relief. Dr. Thomas Hackett, chairman of the Department of Psychiatry of the Harvard Medical School, states, "Trying to separate functional from organic factors in long-standing pain is both vexing and unprofitable." Yet in the practice of medicine, much effort is still made to distinguish "real" from "imaginary" pain. Unintentionally and contrary to better judgment, we have established a hierarchy of body over mind and it has conditioned the way we think about health and disease.

A heart problem, an ulcer, even a broken bone, is intellectually understandable. Emotionally, the feelings are acceptable: "I got sick, there was nothing I could do about it. That's the way things happen." Pain, which has the dual problem of being immeasurable and made up of physical as well as perceptual aspects, is poorly understood as an integrated entity.

Take the case of Karen Talmadge. Karen is a thirty-six-year-old operating room nurse who, up to three months ago, had a mild but chronic back problem that affected her only at night after a long day in the operating room. Usually energetic, spry, and efficient, she began to experience muscle spasms and pain; this problem necessitated a reduction in work hours. She became withdrawn and dispirited. She was shunted from doctor to doctor, but her X rays and myelograms were normal. Her pain persisted, however. She began to question herself: why, with a normal X ray, did she still have pain? Sensing a helplessness on the part of her physician, she began to become ashamed. Caught up in a cycle of shame and anxiety, her pain was magnified and her ability to grapple with that pain diminished. Karen, a trained nurse, would not have questioned the reality of a rash on her arm or a fractured ankle. Because pain cannot be shown to others, though, patients like Karen become guilty and depressed. In extreme situations, patients with pain stop functioning in the working world and contract their social life to one or two people in whom they can confide. To them, the world demands proof, and if no proof is forthcoming, the pain cannot be real.

What Karen and millions like her do not understand is that the absence of proof in the old sense of physical evidence does not mean that pain does not exist. *All pain is real,* whether its effects and causes are demonstrable by our present tools or not. As a matter of fact, a new instrument called a PET (Proton Emission Tomography) scanner promises to show us malfunctioning and perhaps painful areas by taking X rays of *function* rather than of anatomy. Altered pain chemistry can be seen on video tubes with this tool. Although the PET scanner is only a research tool now, within

five years patients like Karen will be able to demonstrate the reality
of what they feel.

QUESTION NO. 2

If My Pain Is Physical, Not Imagined,
How Can Anything
but Physical Treatments Help Me?

Chronic pain is like a five-way intersection. If the traffic flows well
from all directions, the intersection stays clear and getting your car
through is uncomplicated and automatic. However, if one of the
roads leading into the intersection has a broken stoplight and cars
keep feeding into the intersection, then pretty soon it becomes
jammed, uncomfortable, and difficult to get through. Chronic pain
has many roads feeding into it also: physical (injury to a set of back
muscles and ligaments, for instance); emotional (depression magnifies the effect of pain); and behavioral (cleaning the entire house
in one day makes pain worse). These components, and many more,
affect our awareness of pain. An overload in one area jams the intersection and pain becomes worse.

Pain is not felt as pain until it passes from our point of injury (the
back, for example), across the nerves, into the spinal cord, and into
the brain. The brain tells us that the signals it is receiving are "pain"
signals and from where they come. These brain circuits, though, also
intersect with other circuits in the brain—emotional circuits, for instance, and circuits for our senses, and awareness circuits. In the
brain, then, pain signals can become altered and changed. They can
also change us. Thus we can become distracted from pain, depressed
from pain, or angry from pain. Conversely, it is possible to alter the
sensation of pain by changes in our emotional state. There are many
reports of soldiers on the battlefield who have received mortal
wounds, but who did not feel any pain until they returned to their
MASH unit or nearby field hospital. You yourself, I'm sure, have
experienced the distraction of a pleasurable experience blocking out
the perception of pain for a time. The dentist may play soft music to
soften the harsh reality of tooth pain. He, too, is using the body's
ability to change pain by other than physical methods. As Mon-

taigne said, "We feel one cut of the surgeon's scalpel more than ten blows of the sword in the battle."

We are fortunate that emotion, awareness, and other such pathways are part of our pain circuits, for we may then use a whole host of methods for dealing with pain—not just the physical.

QUESTION NO. 3

Why Do I Hurt When It Rains or When I Change My Routine? How Can I Predict When I Will Hurt?

The coverings of the joints, called the synovia, and the coverings of bones, called the periostea, are extremely well innervated: they have hosts of receptors buried in them that detect stretching and pulling and pain. The synovium and periosteum are often inflamed in chronic pain patients. Muscle coverings, or fascia, are tightly bound to the muscle, are well innervated, and highly sensitive to stretch.

Usually, rainy weather is accompanied by falling barometric pressure. It is a physical law that a balloon will expand if the barometric pressure goes down, in an attempt to equalize the pressure inside and outside the balloon. So too with joints, which can be viewed as balloons. When the barometer falls, the synovium expands, tugging on already sensitive tissue and increasing the sensation of pain. Multiply this by all the joints and bursae (fluid-filled sacs placed as cushions where muscles attach to bones) in your body, and you will have some idea of why the weather plays such a tremendous part in your pain.

As a matter of fact, one of our treatment tenets deals with learning what parts of your pain are due to what causes. Although you cannot do anything about the weather, you can benefit from the knowledge that weather is causing the pain and it will be *time-limited:* when the weather clears, the pain will end. The knowledge that something will end is often enough to reduce the anxiety connected with it and thereby reduce the associated muscle tension. This, in turn, decreases pain.

Changes in routine cause adjustments in physical and emotional parts of life. The housewife who must alter her car pool schedule worries that her son will not be picked up on time. This causes fear, which leads to anxiety, which leads to muscle spasm and pain. The executive who must take a sudden trip and is afraid of flying will often experience a flare-up of his pain. We cannot accurately predict when we will hurt, but we can approach accuracy by identifying what stressors (e.g., weather, or flying, or anxiety about children) worsen pain. We do this realizing that these problems are time-limited, and trying to alter their impact on our lives may alleviate and shorten the amount of pain they are prone to cause.

QUESTION NO. 4

Do Pain-Killers Help?

Pain-killers, known medically as analgesics, are useful for *acute* injuries where severe pain lasts only a few days or a week. "Authorities" who tell you that drugs have no use in any pain treatment are simply wrong. Pain-killers are, however, addictive and habit-forming; that is, you can easily build up a tolerance so that, as time goes by, more and more medication is needed to do the same job. We hear comments such as "They just take the edge off" and "They make me groggy but don't do anything for the pain." Indeed, most medications do nothing for chronic pain after a while, and they do affect concentration and awareness. There is very little place for them in the treatment of long-term pain. There is new evidence that suggests that the body is able to produce its own pain medications, called endorphins. Taking pain medications on a long-term basis may well shut off this capacity; consequently, long-term use of these medicines may actually increase pain.

But people are becoming phobic about pain. We are fast becoming a nation unable to tolerate any pain. In America, we grow up reading about pain relievers, whistling catchy jingles, wondering if two Excedrins are as effective as two Anacins or really just as good as one Extra-Strength Tylenol. Will the pain reliever upset my stomach? Should I take some antacids? Is a long-acting spansule preferable? Bewildering? Certainly, but there is no escape. Even the medical journals are filled with advertisements for wonderful new pain relievers.

Pain is big business in America. Even the minor drugs have be-

come a major industry. Twenty thousand tons of aspirin are made
(and presumably consumed) annually. Norman Cousins, who is an
editor and a scholar but not a physician, concisely summarizes
America's enchantment with pain-killers:

> We know very little about pain . . . indeed, no form of illiteracy
> in the U.S. is so widespread or costly as ignorance about pain—
> what is it, what causes it, how to deal with it without panic. Al-
> most everyone can rattle off the names of at least a dozen drugs
> that can deaden pain from every conceivable cause—all the way
> from headaches to hemorrhoids. . . .

Fearing pain, Americans desire to eliminate it from their lives.
Automatically, dentists and physicians will offer pain medication to
a patient in anticipation of the discomfort that may accompany a
procedure or illness, as if the experience of pain were equivalent to
bad treatment. Would a good doctor allow his patient to suffer? Is
the "prevention of suffering" not part of the Hippocratic oath by
which we, as physicians, are bound? Would the public not shudder
to consider the dentist who, after extracting a tooth, adamantly advises his patient to distract himself sufficiently over the next hour to
avoid the sensation of pain and throbbing?

Our practice and others' are rife with patients who have become
addicted to pain medication in the past. The consequences of long-
term use of analgesics are just not worth the little that they do to
quell discomfort. You can learn to control long-term pain better and
more safely than any drug can.

QUESTION NO. 5

If I Must Live with My Pain,
How Can I Learn from It?
Can I Use It to Help Me in Any Way?

It is always difficult to tell a patient to "live with" this or that condition. Our society demands answers and cures which many times
are not readily available. For an answer to this question it is helpful
to turn to two patients who had no hope of removing all pain, yet
were able to use it to advantage in unusual ways.

At one New York City hospital the Cancer Treatment Center

takes up one half a city block. It looks like what it is: a research center designed to probe one of medicine's mysteries. Yet it is also the repository of the hopes and dreams, sorrows and yearnings, of cancer patients and their families. It is charged with both the electricity of scientific discovery and the currents of human emotion.

Pain is a constant companion there, and we learned, as most do who spend any time there, to respect its presence as well as to resent it. As we probed deeper into the quality of life of cancer patients, it became clearer that pain was an experience some of the patients could not and should not do without. Many of the patients were able to manage quite well with a modicum of pain. In a way, to be able to function with pain, and despite it, was a source of pride for these people who had very little control over their own destinies.

Brenda Hillary was a twenty-one-year-old girl who suffered from the spread of a bone tumor called a sarcoma. Her weight loss and nausea had been controlled, and she was struggling to control her pain. Brenda suffered. But she was still able to struggle against the foe that was her old companion—pain. Like enemies who fight each other for years and always draw and disengage, only to fight again, Brenda and her pain sparred, shadowboxed, jabbed at each other, and every so often engaged in a battle so fierce that an observer must think neither could survive. They both did, though, and then they disengaged, to fight again another time. To Brenda, her pain was a sign that she was alive enough to fight. She wasn't numb; she hadn't given up. She didn't want her pain to give up either. For that would have meant numbness, and the next step would be death. The perception of pain was an important part of her life. Again, our appreciation of the nature of pain took on added color as we realized that not only emotions such as depression and sorrow and fear were involved, but also pride and a sense of triumph. Brenda taught us the human dimension of pain.

Kyle Ross needed to learn to use his pain in another way. He was a depressed homosexual man who, on the eve of his fortieth birthday, remorseful because of the loss of his most recent lover, made a serious attempt on his life. Totally inebriated after using a quart of vodka to chase down his residual stash of Valium, he drew a warm bath, disrobed, and emphatically slashed a wrist, severing a radial artery. The unexpecting vessel was so thoroughly traumatized that it responded with a fitful spasm, which was sufficient to prevent the man from bleeding to death. Fortunately, the cleaning woman arrived early, and, discovering the atrocity, she summoned the fire department rescue squad. Brought to the hospital and treated in the intensive care unit, the man recovered and was transferred to our unit for observation and treatment.

At this point you may be wondering what all this has to do with pain. There is a relationship—an important one. We talked with Mr. Ross, finding out where he was born, grew up, attended school, where he worked, and so on. He spoke openly and freely about his life, even his plans for the future. Less than forty-eight hours after trying to end his life, he spoke optimistically about what that life held for him. He was neatly dressed and groomed, patiently awaiting visitors. Even his appetite had fully returned. On the ward he was cordial, talkative, spending time chatting with the patients and staff. When asked about what he had done, he had no recollection of the self-inflicted wounds that brought him to the verge of extinction. He expressed no trace of sadness, remorse, or depression. He was, by his own admission, "over his unhappiness." A bit unsettled by waking up in the intensive care unit hooked to a respirator, watching his heartbeat parade electronically across the face of an oscilloscope, he felt a few days' rest would settle everything back to normal. The only residual of damage was the puff of fluffy white bandage pillowed around his sutured wrist.

How could anyone ravage himself so thoroughly and two days later be well? We felt we had to "do something." Grabbing his chart we worded the note, complete with a diagnosis, "masked depression." Masked, because the classic signs of depression—sadness, tearfulness, loss of appetite, difficulty concentrating and moving— were seemingly absent. We ordered antidepressant medications to be given three times daily. Mr. Ross was going to get well even if he did not know he was sick. The patient never got the medication. Before the nurse could fill our orders, we stopped and tried to reconstruct the problem. "He is depressed; he has to be. Why else would he have butchered himself the way he did?" "Yes, but do you see any evidence of his depression?" "No." "The symptoms are masked." "But there is no depression."

We decided against the antidepressants. The patient *needed* to be depressed. If he could not feel his pain, he would have left the hospital and done the same thing over again. This was, of course, an extraordinary idea and one quite contrary to our ideas of what being a good doctor was all about. It was new to us to think about making someone feel worse as part of an effort to make them feel better. We needed to help him find his pain. It was there; he just didn't know how to feel it. Somewhere in all his struggling to keep things together, he had lost the ability to tolerate pain. He could not accept the pain of aging or tolerate the pain of loss. To consider pain as part of life and find the strength to feel it, to battle against it, is the lesson of chronic pain to learn from this patient. Although not a pain patient, he helped us to understand the components of emotional pain.

In the end, Mr. Ross was able to face his pain, to dissect the causes and components of it. He was also able to discover enough things about himself that he never had to feel suicidal depression again. He was able to learn from his pain, and he recovered completely.

QUESTION NO. 6

What Is There to Understand About Pain? It's a Simple Feeling, Isn't It?

Pain is certainly a feeling, but it's a rather complex one. It carries a message that is personal and profound to the person bearing it. Sometimes decoding that message is a difficult task. It requires patience and understanding. To illustrate, the following is a story of a person who searched for years to understand her pain's message.

Dorothy looked eighty, although she was only fifty-five. She appeared tired and drawn, and although it was early in the morning, she was stooped and bowed with a somber expression, a long face, and dulled, filmy eyes. Perhaps it was a measure of how far apart we were when we first met that she talked incessantly of the lingering, excruciating, incapacitating pain she felt in her amputated arm. Our preoccupation was with the intense sadness that radiated from her every feature and gesture.

Dorothy's left arm had been amputated seven years before because of cancer. She was now free of the cancer, but she was never free of a constant, stabbing, knifelike pain *which she felt in the arm that had been amputated.* The brain still held on to the ghost of the arm, and Dorothy was told by her brain, against her better reason, that the arm was still there.

Dorothy had sought help from internists and neurologists across the country. She was referred to us almost as a last recourse. Dorothy, of course, had practically given up hope, but we talked anyway. She was unmarried, living alone, and managing by herself. She worked as a bookkeeper in a lawyer's office; she lived a simple life of work and then home without many of the other pleasures life has to offer. Her arm gone, she was still able to function on the job, but she felt old and alone and depressed. She sewed with a machine and drove a car, but a strange thing had occurred throughout the last seven years: the phantom of her left arm haunted her. She could feel the arm helping her right arm when she sewed; she could feel it help her other hand drive her car to work. In fact, the pain was the only thing that allowed her to feel that other arm, and feeling that other arm was the only thing that kept her from feeling like a crippled old woman. After two hours of talking, she began to cry— her first cry in two years, and the first sign that she was ready to begin giving up pain as a substitute for feeling worthwhile.

Dorothy's pain began to take a shape and substance beyond agony only when she was able to speak freely, and when we were ready and able to decode what she was saying about its hidden meaning. For Dorothy, pain was not a "simple feeling," but a complex message that took years to decipher.

QUESTION NO. 7

With All the Modern Treatments for Pain, Why Should I Worry About Emotions and Behavior? Can't Science Cure My Pain?

Calvin was a new man. It frightened him terribly. Three months ago a four-pronged electrode had been inserted into his brain. Radio-controlled, it was able to stop his chronic, intractable pain for up to three hours with the mere twist of a dial. It did so because it released a chemical substance called an endorphin, which is the body's own pain pill. Endorphins and methods of stimulating them were discovered in 1977. Newer and more exciting mechanisms of pain relief are continuing to be discovered at a rapid rate. Pathways of pain conduction are being mapped out; connections inside the brain and out are being pieced together. The relationship between the physical, the emotional, and the behavioral have their counterparts in the tiny microinteractions at cellular levels. From the gates that close off pain circuits to the measurement of tolerance, advances are exploding.

Calvin was a marvel of this new technology. Up until three months ago, his pain would rampage out of control for up to thirty-six hours at a time. Now, a true six-million-dollar man, Calvin could turn off the pain effortlessly. He was terrified. It seems that his personality had changed along with his ability to turn off the pain. Once a rowdy mechanic, Calvin had turned into a man who thought before acting, who analyzed and weighed before fighting. He was now feeling anxiety as he weighed and measured; he had become a thinking man rather than an acting machine. But Calvin was no longer *Calvin*. He was—someone else. In the time it took to insert the electrode into his brain, he had traded not only his pain but his personality. He was literally meeting himself for the first time.

Upon consideration, Calvin really portrayed the concept of a pain *system:* his personality, his emotions, his pain, his back, indeed his *identity,* shifted together as a whole, a unit. No clean surgical cut here. No isolated emotional change. Nothing less than total reorganization of a human being's physical and emotional interdependence. We had worked for four years with patients suffering from chronic pain, and we knew, intuitively at first but then through experience, that all parts of a person's life had to change to alter pain. Calvin was the end product of using some fancy electronics and a bit of hardware to do the job, but the principle remained the same.

Science, used alone, can bring about profound changes. Physical advances, however, are only one part of the pain system. As with any system, if you change part A, you must change part B. The behavioral, emotional, and familial parts of pain must also be addressed if an attempt at true pain control is to be successful.

Chapter 2

WHAT IS PAIN?

WHY WE FEEL PAIN

Pain can't really be defined, except by you, the reader. Think of the word. A feeling comes to mind—unpleasant, uncomfortable, irritating, an expectation of danger, anticipation of hurt. One can define it anatomically, physiologically, biochemically, in terms of time, in terms of ergs, in terms of functioning, even in terms of decibels of "ouches." It is a curious thing; it is a universal feeling but each of us feels it differently. One of the difficulties in treating pain is that as universal as this feeling is, it is also the most personal of feelings. No one else can feel your pain. You, then, define the feeling, while we attempt to define the anatomy.

Specialized nerve cells, called neurons, evolved to carry the messages of the body. Some neurons are microscopic, as in the brain. Some are huge: the sciatic nerve is a trunk line almost three feet long. Some are covered with a substance called myelin, like an insulated wire. These carry messages faster than do those neurons which are unmyelinated, or not insulated.

The neurons originate in receptors—specialized endings which can pick up stimuli from the outside environment (temperature and pressure are two kinds of stimuli picked up). Sight is an example of how this works. The specialized nerve endings of the retina are able to receive the messages of photons of light and convert them to sight. Similarly, a certain pattern of reception by a set of specialized receptors also means "pain." This message is then carried through the neurons in the form of electrochemical impulses. Many atoms in the body carry an electrical charge. These atoms are called ions and their movement accounts for the "current" we call nerve impulses.

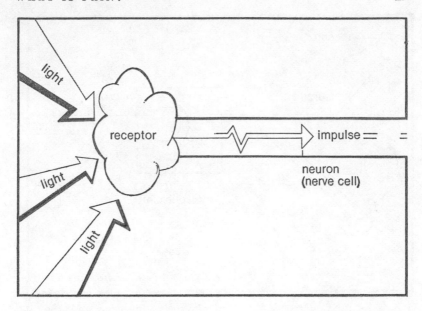

The start of a nerve impulse.

THE IMPORTANCE OF THE CLEFT

The end destination for many of the impulses carried by the neurons is the brain, where the sensation of pain is identified and localized. Before these impulses can get to their destination, however, they must traverse a break in their nerve chain. One neuron ends and another then begins, but they never touch.

They are separated from each other by clefts called synapses. The synapses are bathed in fluid and in order for a message to traverse this chasm a substance called a *transmitter* must be present. The transmitters are complex molecular messengers. There are many different transmitters—acetylcholine, norepinephrine, serotonin—but they must be there in sufficient quantity to act as a bridge between neurons. A transmitter can be altered. For instance, the South American Indian poison curare acts by interfering with acetylcholine and blocks its action, thus paralyzing the victim. In the jungle this is used for survival. When hunting, the Indians of South America dip their arrows in curare. Its paralyzing action can bring death in under a minute, thus ensuring the provision of meat for the tribe. Even in the operating room, survival can be helped by synthetic curare. When injected into a person about to be operated upon, it paralyzes

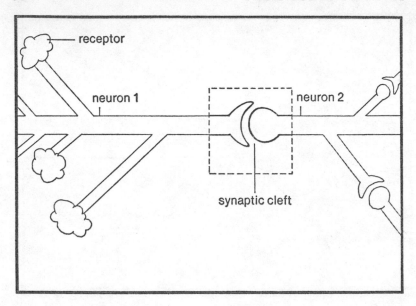

How nerve cells connect.

respiration, allowing the anesthesiologist to breathe for the patient in a more rhythmic fashion.

The cleft is important in other ways also. It has been found that a decrease in the amount of the transmitter norepinephrine causes or is associated with depression. There are drugs called antidepressants which can reverse this decrease and thus prevent depression. Strangely, these drugs also seem to have a beneficial effect on pain. We have known for years that pain and depression were linked. Here is an anatomical reason to tell us why.

The Pathway

Nerve impulses begin in specialized endings called receptors, travel electrochemically along the neuron, across the cleft and continue through another neuron. Most of these messages find their way into the spinal cord and are carried in special bundles of nerves called *tracts* to the brain. In the brain, they pass through any number of areas depending upon the location and utilization and destination of the message. Most of them pass through a structure in the brain called the thalamus where pain is somehow—we are not sure how—recognized as pain and then goes on to localizing receptors.

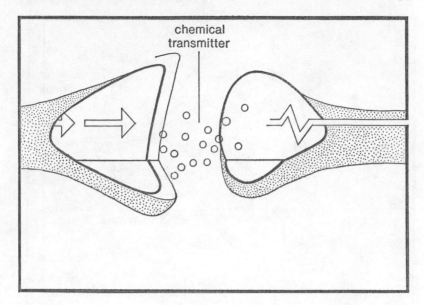

Pain information transmitted between nerve cells across synapse.

In the brain, of course, the messages are acted upon by impulses from many different sources—from the five senses, from depression circuits, and from memory traces called *engrams,* of previous pain experiences. These engrams are memories of how pain affected us in the past. The "color" of pain is altered by these engrams. In much the same way, the color of our pain is altered by our expectations of what that pain will be like. These two factors, engrams and expectation, play a most significant part in our perception of pain. From centers in the brain, pain messages—after alteration by input from the environment, our senses, our memories, and our expectations—are shunted to various centers for processing and action.

The processing and action may take the form of motor action, such as massaging an area that "hurts." It may take the form of oral communication: "I hurt." Most likely, it will emerge as a complex sensation which is uncomfortable, and a complex action involving speech, movement, and, by extension, other people, from family to doctors.

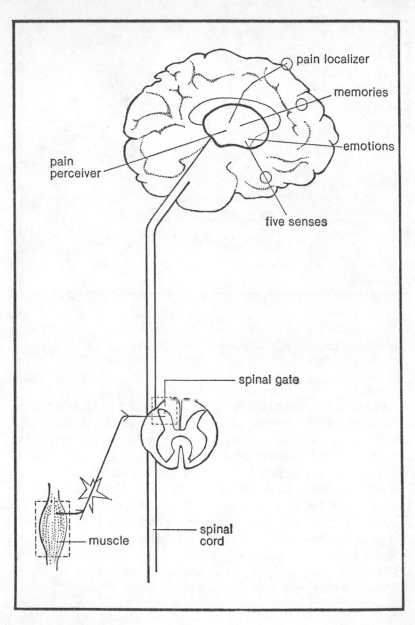

A pain pathway.

DIFFERENT PATHWAYS

We can divide the pathways used for pain messages into three different types: those using reflex arcs, those carrying the message of acute pain, and those relaying chronic pain signals.

Reflexes

Although carrying pain messages, simple reflexes require no thought, because reflex pathways do not involve the brain. Take the example of touching a hot stove. Nature has built into us the ability to react without thinking in those situations where the threat of imminent danger requires immediate action. The threat of a burn requires immediate action in the form of taking our hand away from the stove. It requires no thought, just quick motion. The pain impulses pass very quickly over myelinated fibers (called A and C delta fibers) to the spinal cord. Instead of traveling up the spinal cord to the brain, the impulses are registered by a motor nerve in the spinal cord, which conducts them to the appropriate muscle to withdraw the hand. The perception of pain comes later, thus protecting us from injury first and reminding us afterward how unthinking we were.

Another reflex that involves chronic pain sufferers causes muscle spasm. The pathway of this reflex travels through the skin. Sometimes, if this arc is interrupted, muscle spasm can be aborted. This is important since muscle spasm is thought by some to account for 50 percent of chronic pain. There are several agents, available in spray and lotion form (such as ethyl chloride), which can be used to block this cycle and shut off muscle spasm. As we progress to more complicated forms of pain, the concept of breaking cycles will become even more important.

Acute Pain

Acute pain involves not only the reflex arc but nerves in the spinal cord, the brain cortex (or conscious center of the brain) and the emotional centers in the brain. It, too, has a purpose, as it warns us much like an alarm bell that something is damaged and we had better take care of it. A stubbed toe that hurts for several hours is a good example. The pain of the toe ends. It is finite. How it ends we are not quite sure, but three of the current theories described later in this chapter will begin to explain this "dampening" of pain. Acute pain is helped toward its end by short-term use of medication or massage or heat. The quality of finiteness, having an end, distinguishes acute from chronic pain.

Chronic Pain

Unlike acute and reflex pains, chronic pain serves no useful purpose. It lasts. The pain signals reverberate on and on in the pain pathways; there is no dampening. A reflex occurs to avoid danger even before an alarm bell goes off, much like a sprinkler in a fire. Acute pain is an alarm which is used by the central control mechanism of the body to alert and send help to the damaged area. Chronic pain is an alarm bell that has stuck. It does not serve to warn us of a damaged part that needs attention, it has *become* the damaged part, and it is the alarm bell itself which needs fixing.

WHY DOES ACUTE PAIN BECOME CHRONIC PAIN?

Peter Frankel has sprained his back. He experiences pain, muscle spasm, irritability, soreness, limitation of motion. He may or may not develop a chronic pain system from this injury. What will determine this?

The fibers of the muscles along the sides of Peter Frankel's spine have been torn at the level of the small of his back. The pattern of impulses picked up by these specialized endings, or receptors, begin an electrochemical signal on its way along a neuron. The signal then reaches a cleft, or synapse. It crosses the synapse by stimulating the bulb at the end of the neuron to release a transmitter. The transmitter then crosses the synapse and starts the signal, called an action potential, in the second neuron. This action potential then is transmitted again electrochemically. The transmitter returns to its resting-place in the first neuron to await repetition of its function. The impulse eventually reaches the spinal cord. It enters the cord through the substantia gelatinosa, a jellylike portion of the cord, and is then transmitted up the cord along various long nerves called tracts. These tracts are specialized, some carrying pain and temperature impulses, some position, some vibration, etc. When the tracts enter the brain, the message is conveyed to the thalamus, where it becomes generally and very diffusely "perceived" as pain, and then on to the cortical centers where it will be localized as back pain. Along the way it is operated upon by memories, expectations, the five senses, and a host of other central mechanisms until its final character emerges. It can then be described by our patient as "I twisted my back and now it hurts with a sharp pain that feels like when I twisted it six months ago." Peter Frankel can also say that he is afraid that he will be incapacitated (expectation) because he knows how much pain has hurt him before (engram, or memory trace). He will take certain precautions as indicated by his doctor or his own experiences. Whether the pain becomes chronic or not, however, depends on the entire system, not just his back muscles. It is important to note, too, that if we look at pain as a system, we can intervene in at least seven places:

1. the skin over the muscle,
2. the muscle tear,
3. the nerve,
4. the synapse,
5. the spinal cord,
6. the thalamus and localizer, and
7. all the other modifiers—expectations, engrams, senses, and all the environmental factors such as family, drugs, fitness, etc.

When we treat pain as a system, we give equal weight to all facets of pain: physical, emotional, familial, etc. Arthur, who had had several operations and who suffered from arachnoiditis, an inflammation of the covering of the spinal cord, was sent from doctor to doctor and finally was told that the pain was "in his head." This was as erroneous as when Pamela, who was significantly depressed, was told by her surgeon that she needed her fourth operation because her pain was continuing. In both instances, only one element contributing to pain was considered. Thus, an opportunity for successful treatment of the pain syndrome was missed. We can examine three developments in the area of pain theory which have helped us to understand pain as a system and why acute pain may become chronic.

TWO PAIN PATHWAYS

Until recently physicians and anatomists thought of pain as if it were a simple cause and effect process, with messages traveling at only one speed. According to the old theories a body part, let's say the back, was injured, and this injured part sent messages of pain, over the nerves, into the spine and into the brain. The brain took the raw signals and translated them into the sensation of pain and then told the body where to feel that pain.

Eventually, scientists began to postulate the existence of more complicated systems to account for differences in pain perception in the same individual and to account for the presence of syndromes such as chronic pain. The theories that began to emerge were the first glimmerings of the recognition that chronic pain was something quite different from the neat little package of reflex arc or even the up-the-spine-into-the-brain route.

Fast Pain and Slow Pain

Two different systems of pain transmission and perception have been proposed which help us understand the difference between acute and chronic pain. These two systems are called the *epicritic* and the *protopathic* systems.

The epicritic is the "fast" pain system that accounts for the pain of acute events such as a pulled tooth, a blow to the head, or a laceration. It is sharp and discriminating, can feel and carry the message of a pinprick. Its pain signals are carried to those areas of the brain responsible for quick decisions about what the message is and where it comes from. These signals are carried over nerve fibers that are myelinated, and these fibers carry messages more quickly than the nonmyelinated fibers. The epicritic system developed millions of years after the protopathic system and remained with us because it was necessary for life. It is like the pony express compared to the horse-and-buggy.

The other system, the protopathic, is "slow" and rather more ponderous. It is an old system and is less efficient than the epicritic; it probably allowed an animal to vaguely sense pain rather than localize it. It is carried on uncovered fibers (which makes it slow), and it passes through some rather old and important structures—old in the sense of having evolved early, and important because they deal with basic emotions and survival. These areas are the reticular activating system (RAS), which deals with activation of the organism and response to external threats and stimuli; the periaqueductal gray area, which is interesting because of some new and exciting research indicating that production of pain-killing hormones takes place here; and the limbic system, which deals with such primitive emotions as pleasure, pain, sexual excitement, and thirst and hunger. The protopathic system is also affected by pain engrams—traces of memory of pain experiences derived from childhood that seem to play a part in modifying pain experiences in adults and in making what might otherwise be inconsequential pain into a major syndrome. In theory, the protopathic system provides a neurologic basis for the persistence, intensity, and emotional content that we see in the chronic pain syndrome.

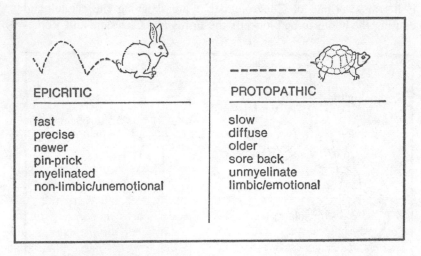

EPICRITIC	PROTOPATHIC
fast	slow
precise	diffuse
newer	older
pin-prick	sore back
myelinated	unmyelinate
non-limbic/unemotional	limbic/emotional

Two pain systems.

The Gate Theory

This theory was postulated by Ronald Melzak and Patrick Wall in 1965. What Melzak and Wall proposed was that the existence of pain is predicated on the presence of a certain pattern of nerve impulses and that the pattern is what determines the amount and localization and the existence of that feeling we call pain. Indeed, they postulated that in chronic pain the protopathic system takes over from the faster, acute epicritic system, and the pattern of impulses usually denoting pain is then carried over into the protopathic system. What we still don't understand is why this happens, but this theory provides us with an anatomic and physiologic model for what we see on a larger level as chronic pain.

The *gate theory* is a provocative model for pain transmission that has allowed us to develop a new method of treatment, the transcutaneous nerve stimulator (TNS). Briefly, the gate theory postulates that there is a gate, or on-off switch, in the pathways carrying pain, in the area of the spinal column called the substantia gelatinosa. According to Melzak and Wall, this gate can be closed down if it gets overloaded. When closed down, it prevents just about all impulses from traveling through it, thus producing analgesia, or the absence of pain. The system is like a tollgate that swings shut when the dispatcher sees too many cars entering the tunnel. It doesn't matter if it's an overload of Chevrolets that are clogging the tunnel and causing the booth to be blocked: the Fords and Chryslers and Volks-

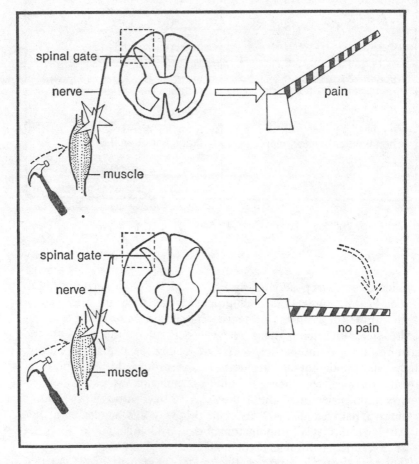

The spinal gate. Any differences between an "open gate" and a "closed gate" are apparently on a cellular level; that is, they are not visible to the human eye without the aid of a microscope.

wagens can't get through either. The assumption was that the gate could be closed down by using an overload of nonpainful stimulus, such as a small electric current, to prevent the pain from getting through. Melzak and Wall's theory seems to hold up, and recent articles have proven its theoretical as well as practical validity.

The Body's Own Pain-Killer

The third and most exciting of the new theories to emerge deals with the body's ability to make its own morphine. In 1975, scientists began to believe in the existence of opiate receptors in the human body; that is, specific targets for the morphine molecule to attach itself to and help quiet pain. In fact, researchers did find such receptors in the brain and digestive system, but at first didn't know what they were. In 1976 other substances called peptides were discovered in the fluid bathing the brain, but their function could not be determined. Then, in 1977, the receptors and the peptides (proteins) were functionally linked. The peptides fit exactly into the structure of the receptors, much like a lock and key. The endorphins (as the peptides came to be known) proved to be connected to the production of the body's own self-made morphine. It seems that the body provides itself with a way of easing its pain without any outside influences. When pain is perceived, the endorphins are activated to dampen that perception. In fact, there is a theory that outside medication shuts off this system, and so by taking drugs for pain we may be defeating the body's own mechanisms for easing its pain. Other fascinating things began to be demonstrated about these endorphins. They seemed to be concentrated in that same periaqueductal gray area of the brain that is associated with chronic pain or protopathic pathways. In addition, Naloxone, a drug that inhibits and reverses the effects of morphine, has in two studies reversed the effect of the body's own morphine. Research currently being conducted indicates that in chronic pain patients on no medication, the effects of externally induced and internally generated pain are made worse by giving Naloxone. Out of this information have come theories that the chronic pain patient is lacking in the ability to make endorphins. Although this idea is controversial and many more studies need to be done, perhaps someday an "endorphin pill"—which could stimulate the body to produce its own natural morphine—will help chronic pain sufferers to cope with their pain more effectively.

A final word on the endorphins. It seems that the adrenal gland also plays a part in producing endorphins. It is the adrenal gland that makes adrenaline, the hormone involved in keeping us ready for danger. It does this when stimulated by ACTH, a hormone produced in the pituitary gland of the brain. It now appears, however, that the ACTH comes from a bigger molecule (called, appropriately, large ACTH), which does give off ACTH, but also produces another molecule when it is cleaved—endorphin.

"Chemically" preparing for pain and stress.

Thus the adrenal glands prepare the body for *danger* and *pain,* so that all efforts can be directed at self-preservation if necessary. Endorphin, in addition to its pain-relieving ability, has profound effects on mood. It has been demonstrated in human studies that high levels of endorphins correlate with a sense of well-being. Three of the elements of our pain system then—depression, the subjective experience of pain, and muscle tenseness in getting the body ready for danger—are all associated with endorphins.

Even newer research being conducted in the field of endorphins within the last year is beginning to demonstrate that endorphins may be released only under *stressful* conditions of pain. To illustrate, we can hark back to our example of soldiers on the battlefield with serious wounds who do not feel their pain until they return to their MASH unit or base hospital. It is almost certain that one of the mechanisms that cause this phenomenon is a release of endorphin. It is appropriate to conjecture at this point that the *stress* of battle and the *stress* of an acute wound are both responsible for the release of that endorphin. Research into this phenomenon continues at various laboratories, where patients are stressed using game theory. Video games can be programmed so that it is impossible for a patient to win. The stress of competitive play without winning seems to produce more pain relief, as reported subjectively and measured objectively by biofeedback, than do nonstressful situations. This has great implications for the future in terms of being able to devise methods of nonharmful stressing, which can trigger a mechanism for the release of endorphins. It may, in addition, be an explanation for the phenomenon of distractability: one is often able to be distracted from pain by stressful situations. It does not, however, answer the question of why pleasurable distractions may also ease the sensation of pain. It is true clinically, however, in our experience, that stressful distractions produce better pain relief than do pleasurable distractions. This is a field ripe for further exploration.

Chapter 3

PAIN ZONES: WHERE YOU HURT
AND WHY

The mind classifies and localizes pain. "My head throbs so badly it will burst" and "My backache is acting up today" are two commonly heard complaints. They are really shorthand. The statement about the head throbbing, for instance, is shorthand for "Intensity and duration of the signals coming from tense muscles and dilated arterioles in my scalp and neck are building quickly. The message that was kicked off along the peripheral nerves has been interpreted by my brain as pain in my head. My husband and I had a fight this morning and I have to get this proposal in to my boss before a twelve-o'clock deadline and this is making the pain worse by increasing tension and knotting up my muscles."

Of course, if you spoke that way, you would soon bore your remaining friends to death and you would be asked to take a long, *long* vacation. So we speak in terms of conditions and regions that hurt and we keep our friends and don't get sent away on long rest cures. This is not an uncommon practice; we often speak in shorthand. For example, "Dinner's on the table, come and eat" does not mean that dinner has by magic just appeared and everyone is invited for a leisurely consumption of the day's offering. It does mean, "I slaved over this stove for two hours cooking this pot roast and making home-baked bread. It's hot now and if you don't turn off the TV and come to dinner this instant you can eat cold mush and I'll just pack up my things and leave." Similarly, if you said this your family would soon be eating each night at McDonald's and you would still be asked to leave for a long, *long* vacation.

The point is that we have developed certain conventions for expressing our wants, needs, desires, and fears in everyday language.

Simple phrases or comments are shortcuts for expressing large ideas. To speak, then, of a backache or a headache is to convey a whole spectrum of ideas and feelings. More often than not, however, our statements are not read correctly by family, friends, or boss. Thus the statement about the headache also says, "I need some relief; push back the deadline," or "I wish my husband understood me better."

As we speak about each of the following medical conditions, remember that these examples are presented with a twofold purpose. First, they present important information about the physical side of chronic pain that will help you to understand better a number of facets of that pain. More importantly, however, remember that the shorthand expressions of pain, like those of other aspects of your life, carry meaning about your emotions and behaviors. You would like to be able to convey these points to the important people in your life, just as with the example about dinner. That is very much what this book is about. Learn the shorthand, understand the physical aspects of your pain, but use this book to fit those aspects into the whole of the puzzle of pain. You will then understand the shorthand and, once that is accomplished, you can convey it to the people who count in your lives.

We have chosen four major pain zones. They are the most commonly encountered, and an accurate base of knowledge about them will help you to understand your specific pain and how to treat it. We have also chosen to include a few special pain problems to illustrate recent clinical advances in the recognition of the causes of pain. Lastly, we have included a brief description of the pain of cancer to illustrate some differences in types of pain, and to point out that mechanisms of pain relief can be derived from many sources.

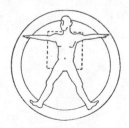

Back zone.

THE BACK ZONE: CIVILIZATION'S PRICE

When human beings learned to stand on two legs they freed their hands for farming and manufacturing and opened the way for back pain forever. The back is the strut which enables us to stand erect. Like a suspension bridge, the muscles, ligaments, and tendons radiating from the spinal column support the erect body, absorbing the tremendous forces generated. As we grow older, or if we weaken one or more of the support struts, the suspension system weakens. Add the factors of age and weakness from injury to our increasingly sedentary life-style, and you have all the elements necessary for the breakdown of this vital interlocking support system.

The vertebral column (backbone) is a column of twenty-four bones which need a force of fifty thousand pounds per square inch to pull them apart, yet are capable of the contortions of an Olympic gymnast. The supporting structures include the ligaments (tough fibrous bands and sheaths which bind the bones), the muscles (large ropelike structures on either side of the vertebral column), and the disks.

What is the disk and why is it so important? The disk is a flat, round wafer with a hard outer shell of cartilage and a gelatinous inner material, much like a flattened liquid-center golf ball. The disks lie between each of the vertebrae of the neck and the upper and lower back. The last five vertebrae are fused into the sacrum, and thus there are no disks in this area.

The disk is the shock absorber of the body. The tremendous forces generated by walking, running, and other forms of exercise are transmitted through the vertebral column. If not for the disks, the bony column would crush itself under its own weight. As a disk ages or is damaged, the hard outer shell becomes "friable"—that is, it begins to break up into small fragments and allows the jelly inside to ooze out. It is this jelly and these fragments which impinge on nerve roots, giving rise to the syndrome called *slipped* (or herniated) *disk*. We should state here, though, that 90 percent of what are called "slipped disks" do not involve any problem with the disk, but affect other structures that make up this vital support system.

The extent of disability from back problems cannot be overestimated. Each of you reading this either has a back problem or knows somebody who does. Seventy-five million Americans have back problems. Seven million new sufferers arise each year and 1.5 million of these new cases are totally disabled either permanently or temporarily. Each year, 200,000 Americans undergo back surgery in the hope, often vain, of cure. Ninety-three million workdays are lost each year to this condition.

A herniated disk is best diagnosed by myelogram, an X ray of the

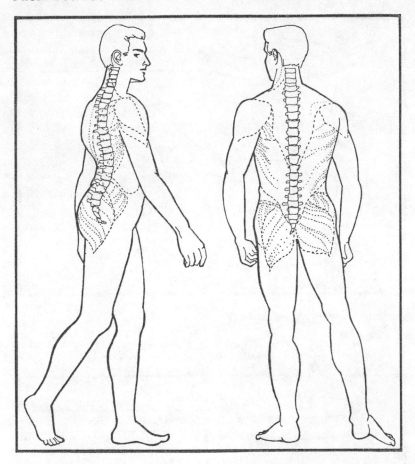

The muscular support of the back.

spinal structures using a liquid metal substance to outline the spinal cord. Other tests to measure the extent of damage from a herniated disk include a diskogram, or direct injection into a disk of the liquid metal substance, and a venogram, an X ray of the disk using the material injected into veins to outline any bumpy patterns in the venous supply. The terms ruptured, slipped, and herniated all refer to the same condition. The disk does not move as a whole, rather, the gelatinous interior begins to protrude or extrude.

If a herniated disk is found, the usual treatment is surgical removal of the disk fragments, although more conservative measures are sometimes taken. A fusion is done when enough material is

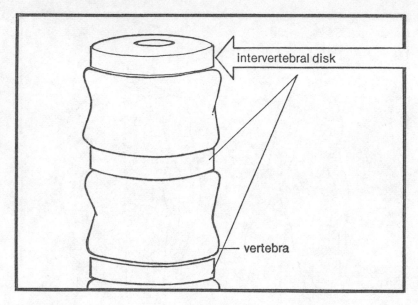

The "shock absorbers" of the back.

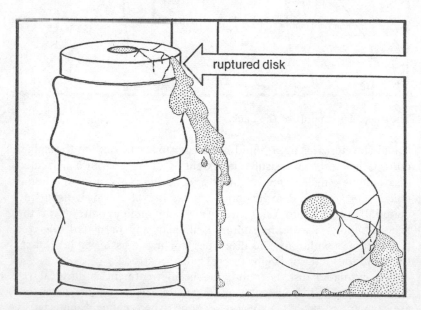

How a disk ruptures.

taken from the spinal column to make it unstable. Vertebrae can be fused together for strength by packing bone chips between them and allowing six weeks for the chips to become a hard, bony bridge cementing two vertebrae. This provides stability without much loss of motion.

Low Back Strain

The major muscles of the back are like two thick ropes extending from the back of the head to the buttocks. Other muscles flare out along the back and buttocks. These muscles all attach at two points on either side of the buttocks called the *posterior iliac spine*. The name is unimportant, except to medical students taking anatomy tests. What *is* important, however, is that underneath each of the ligaments that lead from these ropelike muscles to the bone lies a fluid-filled sac called a bursa. Bursas, too, are cushions. They prevent the rupture of the muscle fibers rubbing over bone from constant friction. They are also, like the disks, shock absorbers, and they are subject to disease. They can become inflamed (bursitis) and cause spasm in the muscles that pass over them. This in turn causes more inflammation and more spasm until a full-blown "back problem" is under way.

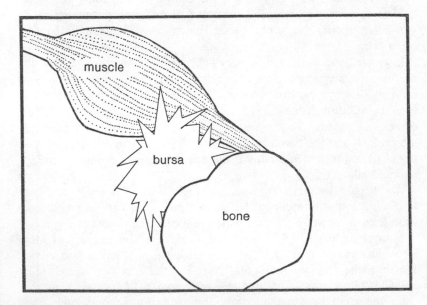

Bursitis.

Initial damage to bursa or muscle is usually mild and transitory, but can become more permanent and part of the chronic pain syndrome. The damage can arise from lifting, or straining, or athletic pursuits. In addition, tension can be reflected in back muscle spasm. The combination of spasm and tension, on top of "splinting" (protecting the injured area by stiffening voluntarily) from the pain, can cause the pain to become worse or spread to the other side of the spinal column. Other stresses can also cause muscle strain. When the weekend jogger limbers up a little too vigorously, he can tear some of the muscle bundles surrounding the spine. These minute tears accumulate and set up an inflammation. The area becomes tender (warning us to stop jogging for the time being) and hot (from the increased blood flow needed to bring the body's healers to the site of injury). The muscle then goes into spasm: it contracts and becomes hardened. This is the body's way of protecting the muscle from further injury. It is difficult to use a muscle in spasm; this is precisely what the body intended, for the muscle needs rest and recuperation. Sixty percent of strains will heal with rest and heat (to increase the blood flow, speeding the flow of endorphins to the site and waste away from the injury). Muscle relaxants can help the pain of spasm, but it is important to let nature do her job by resting voluntarily. Surgery is not the answer to this most common of back injuries. The remedial steps of bed rest, antispasmodics, and anti-inflammatory drugs, plus moist heat to speed healing, will most often help.

Low back strain, though, is very liable to become chronic. Among the numerous causes are poor back maintenance, an already weakened support system, excessive weekend exercise, and improper posture. In addition, frequent (if not severe) back trouble often becomes the focus for vague feelings of physical or emotional discomfort, and the two-headed monster of poor condition and emotional discomfort combine to make this our most common chronic national ailment.

If the pain becomes chronic, relatively new techniques such as biofeedback and transcutaneous nerve stimulation can be employed, as well as the newer medicines which reduce spasm.

Many people swear by a cramp remedy used by trainers of athletes. The chemical ethyl chloride is a topical anesthetic. It deadens the skin when sprayed on it and "freezes" the area onto which it is sprayed. Since muscle cramps involve nerve pathways through the skin, the freezing can sometimes interrupt the nerve signals and break the spasm. It works for some. It does not work for many. For athletes in the heat of competition it may provide a measure of relief. But if it masks an injury it can be dangerous. When athletes play with injured muscles, they often sustain further injury, compounding the original problem. Unless you are being paid to play ball whether injured or not, we suggest you refrain from using ethyl chloride except with your doctor's advice.

The *sciatic nerve* is the largest nerve in the body—three feet long and composed of five roots that combine into one large nerve that travels down the middle of the buttock, down the back of the leg, and into the inner portion of the foot. It often is involved in a herniated disk, because the disks that herniate are usually in the area of these five roots. When this happens, or when the nerve becomes involved without initial disk irritation, we call the problem *sciatica*.

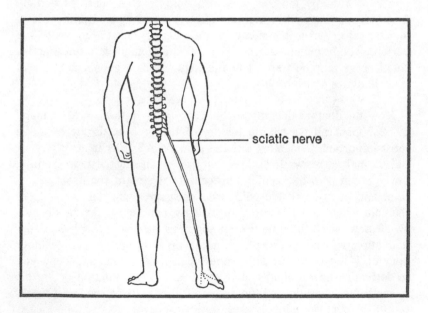

sciatic nerve

The sciatic nerve.

Sciatica is usually described as a knifelike or aching pain along the sciatic nerve, and many patients complain that its pain is worse than the pain of the disk itself. Treatment for sciatica, if there is no disk involved, includes rest and anti-inflammatories, along with mild pain medication such as aspirin, which also helps with the inflammation. If a herniated disk is involved, rest may help temporarily, but other measures, including surgery, need to be considered.

Note that so far in our discussions of treatments, pain medication plays a very small part. We discourage the use of pain medication for more than several days. Most pain patients will agree that medicine of a narcotic nature stops serving its function very quickly, and one is then left with only the addiction and the side effects.

There are many other causes for back pain, including tumors, abnormal bone growth, and congenital defects present from birth (which may not exert an influence until some other element of the support system breaks down).

One problem that has gotten attention lately is the *facet joint syndrome*. The vertebrae, besides being held together by ligaments and supported by muscles, are also held together and aligned by facet joints. On each vertebral body are two flat, disklike plates which project out to the side and smoothly contact the plates of the vertebral body underneath. At times this alignment is altered and a small nerve may be trapped in the joint, causing a pain and spasm that simulates a disk problem.

How do doctors diagnose a back problem if there are so many causes? Generally, a careful history of the problem is the first and most important step. How did the pain begin? Was it an injury or did the pain arise while sitting? The physician must listen carefully, but you can help by keeping an accurate record of the onset, duration, and intensity of the pain, what measures help and what make the pain worse. Your history, surprisingly, can help make the diagnosis 80 percent of the time. Be an educated patient. The physical examination will show the physician if there is spasm and whether your back is tender. He will probe for sensitive areas and bend you to determine how limited your motion is. An examination of muscle strength and sensation of the skin can also help determine whether or not the nerves are involved.

ROUTINE STUDIES

A blood count and urinalysis will help screen for infection and other internal problems remote from but affecting the back. X rays of the back will show any bony abnormalities. Contrary to popular opinion, however, the disks do not show up on regular X rays. One method of telling whether a disk is involved is to measure the spaces between the bones of the back. They should be uniform. If one is smaller, it lends credence to the argument that a disk is involved. Special studies are then recommended.

SPECIAL STUDIES

The myelogram and venogram have already been mentioned. They involve the outlining of structures with dye, and then looking for the presence of unusual patterns in the dye caused by a protruding disk. A diskogram is sometimes done. This procedure is controversial, because it can sometimes further damage the disk. It involves the direct injection of a dye into the disk to outline any problems. If nerves are involved, an electromyogram (EMG) can be done to determine the conduction time in the nerve (the time it takes an impulse to travel from point A to point B). Finally, one of the newest tests to be added to the growing armamentarium is the cone-down computerized axial tomography (CAT) scan. The CAT scanner is an X-ray machine that takes many views of the same plane of the body, and then uses a computer to make a picture that shows all the tissues, instead of just shadows from bones. It gives us a picture much like an anatomical drawing. The cone-down attachment allows us to look at very small areas, and structures as small and difficult to see as a disk.

Trigger Points

There is another problem in the back area that some people encounter: knots that for some reason develop in the neck and shoulders. They are usually associated with stiffness and pain. In addition, they are associated with radiating pain when pressed and consequently are known as "trigger points." Pressure on these knots often triggers pain to radiate along the arm or into the neck or back. Relief of the pain in these knots also seems to relieve the stiffness and pain in other areas. What are these "trigger points" or "knots"?

Muscles are arranged in bundles of fibers. These bundles are covered by a glistening white membrane called the *fascia,* which gives strength, shape, and support to the muscles. At times, and for reasons we really do not understand, local areas of muscle and fascia "knot up," become inflamed, and cause the rest of the muscle to contract, or go into spasm. Sometimes nerves become trapped between these contracting muscles, and it is this pressure on muscles and nerves that causes the radiation of the pain.

What can you do at home to relieve the pain and stiffness caused by these knots? One of the simplest yet most effective methods of pain relief is a special type of pressure directed at the knot, which tends to "flatten" it and bring relief from stiffness and radiation.

First, you should have a partner. You, as the pain patient, cannot exert enough force to flatten the knots. You must, however, be able to point directly with one finger at the knot so your partner does not have to find a needle in a haystack. The knots feel "doughy"; sometimes they are associated with a gravelly or gritty feeling, as if there were pebbles in the knot. The knots may be solitary or multiple, but usually they appear in the same spot each time they return. The trick to flattening the knots is to use the pad of the thumb. Have your partner place his or her thumb pad directly over the knot and, with a circular motion, flatten the knot. He or she may have to dig under the knot or roll it back and forth, but after two to three minutes the knot should disappear. The partner should be careful not to exert too much force, as it is the length of time of the rolling motion rather than the force exerted which will flatten the knot. Deep breathing during the process should help; inhale before the pressing, and as your partner presses, exhale slowly. With the knot's disappearance should come at least temporary freedom from the stiffness and the soreness of the trigger-point pain.

THE HEAD ZONE: "AN HOUR OF PAIN IS AS LONG AS A DAY OF PLEASURE"

English Proverb

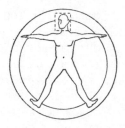

Head zone.

Audrey knew that the pain would come later. Sitting at her desk, the flashes of light in her right eye prevented her from seeing well.

There began that feeling in her stomach that started out as a "sensation" and ended up as nausea and vomiting. She felt ill now and the throbbing on the right side of her head and behind her right eye grew more intense as the minutes wore on. Unable to see, too nauseated to work, and too pained to concentrate, she excused herself and left, asking a friend to drive the two miles to her home for fear of an accident. She stayed home from work for the next two days while her migraine headache sapped her strength and spirit.

It would be a rough conference with upper management. His ideas for the new plant, over which he had labored for months, were in the balance. Indeed, his future with the company would be determined in the next hour. As time passed, he noticed a tightening sensation at the base of his skull and the back of his neck. He had noticed it in times past when he was tense. Slowly the tightness at his neck spread like a band around his head. The band tightened and his head throbbed with the misery of a muscle tension headache. Quickly swallowing some medication recommended for his headaches by a physician, he hoped that he would remain alert enough and had caught the pain early enough to be able to present himself and his work well. He was intensely worried about his career. Of course, this made his headache worse.

These anecdotes are composites, but they do represent the typical picture of developing symptoms in two of the three most common headache syndromes.

This year, 10 to 20 percent of Americans will consult a physician with headache as their primary symptom. Six out of every hundred people experience headaches severe enough to interfere with daily activities. Headaches are persistent and aggravating. Often, they are the cause of partial and permanent disability.

Close to 98 percent of all headaches are caused by one or a combination of two syndromes: muscle contraction and tension, or vascular and migraine.

Muscle-Contraction, or Tension Headache

Muscle-contraction or tension headaches are the most common. It has been estimated that 80 percent of the adult American population suffers from them. This type of headache is most often on both sides, and is described as aching, squeezing, or bandlike, especially in the muscles in the back of the head and the forehead. It often spreads to the shoulders and neck. The scalp is usually tender and there may be spasm or tender nodules around the neck muscles. Slight nausea may be present. Most last only a few hours, although some persist for weeks, months, or even years. Women outnumber men by three to one.

As the name implies, tension is a major cause, as in our illustration of the businessman. The problem is chronic and tenacious. People prone to this type of pain tend to express tension as muscle spasm and tend to experience this spasm in the muscles of the neck and scalp. The underlying tension must be dealt with or the problem will continue and the frustration of chronicity will add to the discomfort.

In our illustration, our businessman was prone to tension headaches in situations where he was acutely anxious. Many of these "spot" situations cannot be avoided. In dealing with the tension, however, there are changes that one can make that can shift the burden of tension away from the head. Also, it is important to understand that the drugs that are often prescribed for chronic tension headaches often dull one's ability to cope as much as the headache does. Used judiciously, they are useful for the short term. But they are all too often used to excess.

Vascular and Migraine Headaches

Vascular headaches also affect women three times as often as men, but they occur in only 9 percent of the population, and children make up one quarter of that 9 percent. Whereas tension accounts for 71 percent of all headaches suffered, 27 percent are vascular. Symptoms usually occur on one side of the head, with throbbing pain often in the temples and the front of the head for a period of hours to days. Classic migraine headache is always vascular in nature preceded by transient neurological symptoms such as flashes of light, strange sensations, body distortion, lightheadedness, or alterations in mood.

Vascular headaches tend to run in families. In women these headaches may be associated with the menstrual cycle or other hormonal changes, but in fact any stimulus, from an emotional upset to a blow to the head, can set them off. There are some patients in whom food allergies or sensitivities, especially to cheese, chocolate, or red wine, will set off a headache.

In practice, headache is still a mystifying disease. Although physicians are learning more about its treatment, the *reason* that human beings seem to be so susceptible to pain in the head is simply not known. Back pain is troubling, but a reason for the breakdown and sensitivity of the back can be found in our evolution from four-legged hunter to two-legged hominid. No such justification can be made for headache. The chronicity of headache pain, then, is made even more frustrating because of this lack of justification. There also exists a certain sense of helplessness in dealing with headaches. Treatment can be efficacious, but prevention is very difficult and it is in this area that the future lies. We do know, however, that headache tends to run in families, and that tension can affect both the muscle-contraction and the vascular headache.

THE FACIAL ZONE: TMJ AND FACIAL PAIN

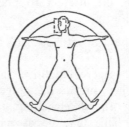

Face zone.

Sarah Gaub arrives in her dentist's office with a list of complaints that include a clicking or popping sound when she opens her mouth widely; a ringing or buzzing sound in her ears; and an aching in the side of her head, over the eyes, and in the back of the head that radiates into the neck and shoulder. She has experienced occasional dizziness and notes that she at times awakens in the morning with her teeth aching, tightly clamped together, and with a soreness at the corner of her lower jaw.

Gloria Kristel presents her physician with a history of headaches occurring over an eight-year period, virtually every day. She is now depressed, no longer being able to deal with the daily discomfort. It is interfering with her relationship with her husband and her children, and she has been to a dentist, a neurologist, a neurosurgeon, a psychologist, a psychiatrist, and an orthopedist. She has had virtually every known neurological testing program, all of which have proved negative. She reports that she is at the end of her ability to cope, is emotionally drained.

Carl Tipton reports to his internist that he is having neck and shoulder pain on his right side and notices occasional headaches involving the right side of his head. Occasionally, he gets a feeling of pressure or discomfort from his right ear. His jaw tires easily when chewing.

All of these patients have described variations of Temporomandibular Joint Dysfunction. This joint is what hinges the lower jaw to the skull. (What we think of as the upper jaw is actually a part of the skull.) The incidence of this dysfunction is higher in women than in men, and those who suffer with it generally are selfless, responsible persons who are chronic worriers.

There are three classes of causative factors in any TMJ Dysfunction. In any given patient, these factors vary in their importance, but, generally speaking, all interact to play a role in producing symptoms. The factors are:

1. Pathological mechanical stresses in the biting relationship (malocclusion).
2. Habit patterns. These are repetitive movements and positionings of the lower jaw outside the range of normal, functional, positions (grinding of teeth, clenching, nail biting, etc.).
3. Emotional Stress. This may be associated with either long-term, deep-seated problems or problems of an everyday social, financial, interpersonal-relations nature.

Pathological mechanical stresses in the biting relationship result from an alteration in the way in which the teeth interdigitate in either a closing position or in a side-to-side movement of the lower jaw. This can happen as a result of losing a tooth, with subsequent tilting and drifting of adjacent and opposing teeth, or after a filling or a bridge is placed in the mouth and does not conform to existing function. These malocclusions can also be due to irregularities in the shape of the dental arches, or can be the result of post-orthodontic imperfections.

The important thing to understand is that, in any of the above circumstances, the muscles that are responsible for the movement of the lower jaw are forced to torque the jaw into an unnatural closing or side-to-side movement in order to achieve the desired jaw position or movement. This means a need for continued extra muscle activity just to perform usual, normal jaw movements. Continued repetitive demands on muscle activity can cause muscle spasms, felt by the patient as pain and soreness distributed according to those particular muscles involved.

Unusual habits concerning jaw movements or positions are generally an expression of a stress. The most common habits include clenching and grinding of teeth, lip and cheek biting, placement of foreign objects (pipes, pens, pencils, etc.) between the teeth, chewing of ice, and nail biting. The degree of their effect depends on the frequency of performance and the intensity of the forces exerted in the jaw movement or position. Hundreds of pounds per square inch can be applied during some of these habits, sending the involved muscles into spasm, and creating pain. Additionally, excessive forces on the teeth and their supporting bone can create loosening of the teeth, wearing down of the enamel surface, and destruction of the bone that supports the teeth in their sockets.

Many of the habit patterns mentioned result in heavy stresses being placed on the muscles of the jaw, as the jaw may be held in extreme positions. These forces are transmitted into the temporomandibular joint itself, and can cause pathological changes in the joint contents. This pathology can then itself alter jaw movements to produce additional muscle spasms and further pain.

Emotional stress acts to create muscle hyperactivity. Stress alone can cause all of the TMJ symptomatology mentioned at the outset of this chapter without the habit patterns or malocclusion being factors. Stress also acts by promoting the need for habit patterns as an outlet, an escape valve. It increases the intensity of the contraction of the muscles during the habit application and does not give the patient an opportunity to allow the muscles time to rest, to reduce the strain on them. Frequently, the patient exhibits a close relationship between periods of pain and periods of heightened stress cycles.

TMJ dysfunctions are generally classified according to their presence either within the joint itself (enclosed by a capsule) or external to that structure (muscles, fascia, etc.). Within the joint itself, such problems as fractures, rheumatoid arthritis, osteoarthritis, tumors, bone spurs, and ankylosis (bony fusions) can occur. Outside of the joint, pathology can include dental pain, sinusitis, muscle spasms, vascular inflammations, muscle inflammation, and other sources. Many times a peripheral problem can cause a problem within the joint. An example of this is the patient with the sensitive tooth on the left side. He starts shifting his chewing pattern onto the right side. Over a period of years abnormal wear patterns on the teeth cause a further shift in joint function. The constant long-term alteration of the biting function results in muscle spasms. The spasms affect the patterns of jaw movement which, in turn, create problems with the joint space itself.

A thorough, detailed history is the first step in the diagnosis of any temporomandibular joint dysfunction and its differentiation from the other various disorders causing head and neck pains. Many times, various radiographic or blood studies are necessary to determine the nature of the disorder.

Treating temporomandibular joint disorder involves managing all three of the causative factors, 1) Malocclusion, 2) Habit patterns of jaw movements, and 3) Emotional stress.

Generally speaking, the utilization of a custom-made appliance on the upper teeth can eliminate the effects of malocclusion and of jaw-movement habit patterns. These appliances are generally worn twenty-four hours a day. When the mouth is closed, the biting surface of these appliances contacts fully with all of the lower teeth. There is no need for the patient to torque the lower jaw to gain comfortable contact. In addition, because of the way in which the biting surface is shaped, complete freedom of side-to-side and protrusive jaw movements is secured, vastly decreasing isometric muscle contraction. This freedom of movement diminishes the effects of clenching and grinding habits. In addition, chewing fingernails, pencils, cheeks and lips is all but impossible.

As muscle spasms decrease, symptomatology (pain, clicking and popping of the lower jaw, limited opening movements) decreases. Generally, no alteration to the biting relationship of the teeth is performed until the patient has been free of symptomatology for an eight- to twelve-week period. At that point, whatever method is indicated to achieve the proper biting relationship is instituted. This may involve minor changes in the shape and form of the jaw by means of restorative techniques, or orthodontic repositioning of the teeth.

Management of the emotional stress factors should begin during early stages of treatment. In most cases, no long-term solution to the chronic pain problem involving the temporomandibular joint can be achieved unless the emotional stress contribution is resolved. Therapeutic approaches include utilizing such methods as biofeedback, hypnosis, postural therapy, physical exercise, physical therapy, acupressure, acupuncture, and psychotherapy.

It is important to remember that unless all of the causative factors are addressed, hope for success is limited. As with all complex dysfunctions and chronic pain syndromes, a certain minority of cases do not respond to treatment, despite the clinical expertise of the group directing the therapy. The goal in these cases is to modify the perception of the pain so that adequate function is obtained and the level of quality of the patient's life is raised.

THE JOINT ZONE: ARTHRITIS

"When I walk my hip pains me so greatly that I need to stop and rest and catch my breath every few steps. The pain feels like two raw stones grinding against each other."

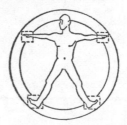

Arthritis zone.

Pain is the most common complaint among the 16 million arthritis patients in this country. The term arthritis literally means inflammation of a joint. The syndrome we think of, however, when speaking about arthritis is the painful, sometimes deforming, even crippling affliction of joints and the muscles and coverings around those joints.

Although there are many types of arthritis (over a hundred), the two types we see most often are called osteoarthritis and rheumatoid arthritis. Osteoarthritis is a disease that affects older individuals much more frequently than younger. Often called "wear-and-tear" arthritis, it is characterized by pitting and roughening of the smooth cap over the ends of long bones (thigh or arm or leg). This cap is called the articular cartilage. In the normal young adult, it is a smooth, glistening, shiny cap that serves as a lubricated, almost siliconelike surface over which the two bones comprising a joint can glide. It prevents bone from rubbing against bone. It is the erosion of this cap and the mechanical wearing of one bone over the other that we feel so painfully. Men and women are nearly equally affected. Recent studies show that both hereditary factors and envi-

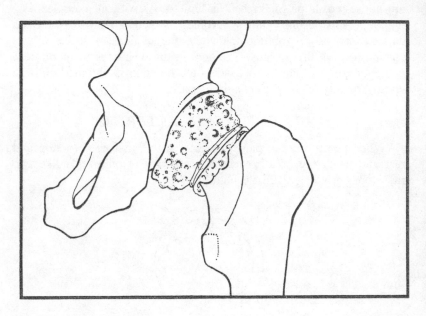

Painful arthritic hip joint.

ronmental factors (excessive use, trauma) contribute to increased
susceptibility.

The disease is ubiquitous. Judging from X-ray findings, over 40
million Americans suffer from this illness, although only one eighth
are affected clinically. This type of arthritis has been found in Nean-
derthal remains (30,000 B.C.) as well as in a variety of animal spe-
cies, including dinosaur skeletons (200 million B.C.).

The symptoms of osteoarthritis are referrable to the joint involved. They include morning stiffness, joint pain, tenderness, and
swelling. There is particular stiffness after periods of rest and aching
in inclement weather. The treatment of osteoarthritis consists of pain
relief, restoring the functions of the joint, and prevention of disability. It is helpful to know that this disease does not become widespread and is usually limited to a few joints. Rest is important; support (cane or crutch), heat, and exercise to avoid muscle wasting all
help. Aspirin for pain relief is often prescribed, but drugs usually
play a minor role in relief of this arthritis since it is not inflammatory. Although cortisone can be injected directly into the joint (and
this may help for a few weeks), it is to be avoided on a regular

basis, as it may accelerate the degenerative process. Surgical procedures include fusion, and great strides have been made in artificial joint replacements for the knee and the hip, and somewhat less successfully so for the shoulder and the elbow.

Osteoarthritis, it has been said, starts the day we are born. Although the wear and tear of arthritis contributes to the erosion of joints, there are other theories suggesting that slow viruses (viral infections that over decades accelerate the arthritic process) may contribute to the susceptibility of certain individuals to this disease.

The second major arthritic illness is rheumatoid arthritis. Rheumatoid arthritis is an inflammatory disease. That is, it involves the structures surrounding the joint and, as opposed to osteoarthritis, is accompanied by inflammation of the synovium, the covering of the joints. That is why it often presents with red, hot, painful, inflamed joints. Rheumatoid arthritis may be a part of a general order of arthritis called *autoimmune diseases:* that is, the body becomes allergic to itself and causes reactions in various joints and the surrounding tissue. Other diseases in this group include systemic lupus, polymyositis, and scleroderma (where the skin becomes hard and constrictive). Rheumatoid arthritis affects women more than men and epecially women between the ages of twenty and forty. It can often be a crippling disease because of the weakening of the tendons, ligaments, and other structures that support the joint. Laboratory tests—particularly tests measuring proteins and abnormal antibodies—are very helpful in diagnosing this condition. Your doctor may order tests called ANA, complement fixation, and anti-DNA, all of which are directed toward telling us whether the body is attacking its own cells.

Treatment depends on the severity of the disease. Aspirin is the mainstay in mild to moderate rheumatoid arthritis, because of its pain relief and anti-inflammatory effect. Other helpful drugs include the steroids (cortisone); the nonsteroid anti-inflammatories, such as Motrin; and gold salts. Surgery may play a major role in correcting deformity caused by this disease. For instance, major strides have been made in the production of the implantable knuckle. This joint is often affected by rheumatoid arthritis, and it is important to note that the crippling effect of rheumatoid arthritis on hands could be corrected by implantation of artificial knuckles.

Other forms of arthritis are frequently encountered. The age-old gout, where uric-acid crystals are deposited in joints, is so painful that the mere presence of a sheet resting on the joint usually is enough to cause severe pain. Arthritis may be due to infection, heredity, tumors, sickle-cell disease, hemophilia, etc. It is a most common and, at times, most frustrating cause of chronic pain.

SPECIAL PROBLEMS

MYOFASCIAL SYNDROME

This newly named problem involves the binding down of muscle fibers to their coverings, which are called fasciae. You may have noticed the fascia of muscles when you eat steak. It is the glistening white, tough membrane covering large surfaces of the meat. Similarly, all of our muscles are covered with this fascia. Often, after trauma or for other reasons, the muscles bind to the fascia and inflammation sets in. This binding most often occurs in the neck, shoulder, and upper back areas. The treatment of myofascial syndrome employs heat, anti-inflammatories, and trigger-point injections. These are injections with novocaine alone or in combination with cortisone to break up the knot and reduce the inflammation, easing the binding and the pain. The origins of this syndrome are still subject to controversy, but we know that its effects can range from mild discomfort to incapacitating pain. It can become a chronic illness which recurs and limits the ability to engage in many activities.

TENNIS ELBOW

Tennis elbow is common and painful and does not necessarily come only from playing tennis. It is properly called lateral epicondylitis, but it is fondly known to many as "that ※$※$@%※ elbow of mine." It is responsible for more wins by default in tennis than all the rainstorms the world has known and it is highly resistant to treatment.

Anatomically, the muscles on top of the arm that control the pulling back or extension of the fingers have their ending in a tough, fibrous band of tissue called a tendon. This is fastened to the outside bump above your elbow, called the lateral epicondyle. Tennis elbow is an inflammation of this tendon and the bursae (fluid-filled sacs) underneath the tendon. The inflammation is due to repeated mechanical stress, so early correction of the mechanics that are causing the stress may help to alleviate the inflammation. Many treatments have been tried, from elastic supports to TNS (transcutaneous nerve stimulation see pages 283–84) to surgery.

All in all, these therapies do not work well. If you find you have the problem, rest the arm in a sling and use hot soaks. Injections of steroids and novocaine sometimes help. See your doctor. Swearing does not help but may make you feel better.

REFLEX SYMPATHETIC DYSTROPHY

A fascinating and newly recognized syndrome, sympathetic dystrophy is a disruption of the sympathetic nerves in an extremity.

There are two kinds of peripheral, or outer, nervous systems. The first is the "voluntary" nervous system, which moves the muscles of our body and which we can consciously control. The other is called the autonomic nervous system and has two parts: the sympathetic and the parasympathetic. The autonomic nervous system controls such things as digestion, perspiration, and the muscular action of the heart, bladder, and small arteries (thereby determining their size). These functions are out of our conscious control.

Orthopedic surgeons are accustomed to seeing the sympathetic (nonvoluntary) nervous system disrupted by fractures and immobilization in casts. Often, after a cast is removed, the injured area is warm and red, sensitive to the touch, and subject to a burning sensation. Although the healing time varies, the symptoms will generally disappear after eight weeks or so. We are now recognizing a similar set of symptoms in patients with back pain, and the theory proposed to explain this is that the sympathetic nerves have been damaged—just as if a limb had been broken and placed in a cast, but without that visible cause—in a manner we don't yet understand. This is an extremely important finding, for if a patient with back and leg pain suddenly complains of burning pain, it is most often due to sympathetic dystrophy.

This form of sympathetic dystrophy generally does not heal on its own, and there are currently two forms of treatment. At times a small operation to sever the sympathetic nerves can be performed. This procedure produces some instability in the limb's reaction to heat and cold, but may eliminate the pain problem. More recently, however, it has been found that an injection of novocaine and a steroid into the spinal canal will help to alleviate or even eradicate the problem. We will go into the mechanisms of the spinal block in a subsequent chapter.

PHANTOM LIMB PAIN

In this fascinating but hazily understood pain syndrome, patients who have had an extremity amputated still feel the amputated extremity as if it were present. Sometimes, as we have discussed, the reasons for this are rooted in an emotional issue. But there are also physiological causes. The brain, which localizes and perceives pain, still has the representation of the limb stored in its memory. The limb is then "perceived" to be still present. The sensation of pain can be independently produced and perceived in circuits in the brain. It can then be felt to be present and as real as if the limb were still there. This gives credence to our theories that pain messages need not originate in an affected area and serves to make the conception of pain as a system with many interdependent parts even more firmly established.

CANCER PAIN

Though we often hear of the terrible pain of cancer, many types of cancer are curable, and its pain, consequently, is of limited duration. The pain of a tumor, even in those incurable cases, is often less severe and intractable than is expected by both patient and doctor. Much of the pain of cancer is caused by direct pressure of the tumor on vital structures such as nerves and organs. Radiation, chemotherapy, and surgery can all help to remove the source of pain by helping to shrink the tumor and relieve pressure. Methadone, a drug used in the treatment of morphine and opiate withdrawal, has been successfully used in the treatment of cancer pain. Even in those cases in which the cancer cannot be cured and the pressure and infiltration of the tumor is an insoluble problem, it is essential to give the patient a choice of treatment using a judicious amount of narcotics but utilizing also the newer techniques of behavioral modification, relaxation therapy, self-hypnosis, and mechanical devices such as the transcutaneous nerve stimulator (see pp. 283–84). Those cancers which are treatable by surgical or radiologic methods show dramatic responses in reduction of pain.

Finally, the emotional components of pain—dependency, fears of abandonment, anger, and isolation to name a few—are very much heightened in the arena of cancer, where the fear of a possibly fatal disease speeds the perception of pain and can magnify it. If these psychological issues are successfully addressed, they can contribute markedly to successful pain reduction.

Pain and cancer are not synonymous. Many cancer patients remain pain-free during their treatment. Many others feel minimal pain. For that group in which pain is a major factor in the course of their illness, the balance of the correct analgesia; surgical, chemical, or radiological shrinking of the tumor; and the use of the newer pain therapies has brought significant relief.

Chapter 4

GETTING CAUGHT ON THE
PAIN-GO-ROUND

Joan Blaylock is a thirty-two-year-old legal secretary. For the past two years, she has been caught in the cycle of chronic pain. Her plight began innocently enough when she slipped off the third rung of a stepladder, twisting her neck and shoulder as she fell. Initially unscathed, she later developed headaches and radiating pains in her arms which have persisted since shortly after the accident.

Immediately after the injury, Joan's family physician suggested a week's bed rest. The pain got worse. He increased the dosage of pain relievers and muscle relaxants. Still her pain persisted. Three weeks after the injury, she consulted an orthopedic surgeon who recommended physical therapy and diathermy (heat therapy). Encouraged by his assertive attitude, she religiously attended her therapy. In fact, she tried to be the model patient, pushing herself to do as much as she possibly could. Unfortunately, nothing seemed to help. After three months of physical therapy, she was still unable to return to work, felt extremely uncomfortable lying in bed at home, and was absolutely convinced she had cancer—and that no one was willing to tell her.

Her pain persisted. Referred from one specialist to another, she was treated with all forms of heat, whirlpool, even biofeedback. Her pain got worse. She missed her job. Sitting at home watching too much television and having little useful work to occupy her mind was ruining her concentration. Reading the morning newspaper became a chore. She lost interest in current events, sports; even her passion for bridge was dulled. Fortunately, her accident occurred on the job and so workmen's compensation helped defray her costs and expenses.

Despite the most potent pain medication, regular physical therapy, and seemingly endless bed rest, medical treatment failed to produce lasting relief. Whenever she began to feel a slight bit better something would happen to trigger a setback. Then it would start over— ten days of bed rest, regular doses of pain-killers and muscle relaxants, and more boredom. Swallowing pills became automatic. With consternation, she noted her tolerance for Percodan (a narcotic pain reliever) had dramatically increased.

After eighteen months of chronic pain, a series of events occurred that greatly affected the course of Joan's recovery. A lifelong battle against overeating, which for many years had been controlled by strict diet and frequent exercise, once again became an unmanageable problem. She gained forty pounds. Her slender figure, once a source of pride and self-esteem, was now hidden in a fat, unattractive body. What was left was a closet filled with lovely clothes three sizes too small. As her self-esteem plummeted, so went her confidence. She felt helpless and depressed, and her headaches became even more intense and persistent.

As physical therapy provided only minimal relief, she stopped going. She became lackadaisical, if not blatantly indifferent to her physicians' recommendations. Gradually, subtle accusations that she was exaggerating her discomfort were voiced by her physicians, who balked at her resistance to physical therapy and the constant demands for pain medication. Following a particularly caustic blowout, the neurologist treating her headaches refused to renew a narcotic prescription, stating, "Joan, your need for medication is out of proportion to your pain. You are abusing the drug."

Joan was furious. Feeling victimized, she accused the doctor of heinous insensitivity as well as not understanding a damn thing about pain. As the volume of her verbal assaults increased and the number of expletives escalated, the neurologist became overtly cautious and made it clear he would not prescribe any more pain medication. Obviously uncomfortable with this outspoken belligerent woman and her irresponsible accusations, he sternly (and almost punitively) advised her to seek psychiatric help for her drug addiction. Joan blew up. Here she had this awful persistent pain and this doctor was sending her to a psychiatrist—as if she were crazy.

The blowout with the neurologist fractured Joan's façade of facile cooperation. She was vulnerable and her hurt began to show. After cooling down, she reluctantly accepted the neurologist's suggestion and made an appointment with us, ostensibly to discuss her pain problem.

She arrived no less than thirty minutes late for her initial appointment. Obviously defeated, her childish acquiescence created a tense, mildly hostile climate.

Was Joan's pain imaginary? Did the absence of an organic basis for her pain mean she was mentally ill?

Entering the office, she stared at the floor and without benefit of an introduction began: "Dr. Martin [her neurologist] suggested I come to see you. I have a pain in my neck and constant headaches. I've had it for two years; nothing seems to help."

After a pause she continued: "As ridiculous as it sounds, if I could break my back to have something to show them [the doctors], I would do it. Every time they send me for another X ray, a part of me actually hopes they'll find something—a fracture, a displacement, an infection, even a tumor—just so I could show them that my pain is real.

"I don't blame Dr. Martin for sending me here. He's put up with a lot over the years. Sometimes I don't know how he could stand me. I called so often. He tried his best, but like he said, the medical profession could only do so much.

"After all he had done for me, I could have refused when he insisted I make an appointment to see you. I know the pain is not in my head." Suddenly looking up, gaining eye contact for the first time, she exclaimed, "My God, I could never imagine anything this terrible. I know I'm not crazy!"

"Is that why you think Dr. Martin sent you, because he thinks you're crazy?"

After a slight pause she replied, "No, he's too good a friend. He wouldn't have sent me unless he thought you could help."

For over two years, she had tried to cope with persistent pain. Depression and medication abuse were now part of the problem. As if she were caught in quicksand, the greater the struggle, the deeper she sunk. The thought of seeing a psychiatrist was unbearable. Her argument with Dr. Martin only confirmed what she already knew: she was becoming emotionally ill. Although frightened and a bit overwhelmed, she rather stoically confessed, "Being sick, living in pain is bad enough, but being thought of as a sick person infuriates me. . . . I hate it. . . . After all, I'm really a healthy person."

Joan would go on to effectively eliminate her drug problem and get control of her pain. Once the initial shock of admitting how much of a problem is created as a consequence of *living with pain* and not just because she had pain, she quickly took measures to adjust and adapt. Joan wanted to help herself, and in the end, after handling her embarrassment, she managed to let us offer some therapy.

Inadvertently, Joan had developed a chronic pain syndrome. Like many other people, she desperately wanted to help herself but did not quite know where to begin. Such confusion, created by the frustration of living with pain, is the force that moves the pain-go-round.

GETTING STARTED

Confronted by the emotional agony of people with chronic pain, we recognize the multifaceted problems of patients with physical pain. As we, in our own practice, have become familiar with these complex emotional and physical factors, we have tried to engage people earlier in the course of their illness, before they've exhausted medical resources and received the label of being "psychiatric" patients. Eschewing labels has reaped rewards: no one likes being thought of as nutty, especially when they have real pain. Creating a role for the psychiatrist was not simple; nonetheless, we have found a function integrating psychological with physical therapy for individuals with chronic pain problems.

For the patient suffering with pain the scope of available treatment is extensive and diverse. While we have found no panaceas or miraculous cures, we have found that many forms of treatment have significant value when appropriately administered and applied.

The problem is orchestration and implementation. Many people with pain fail to get it all together. Treatment protocols range from unnecessarily complex to nonexistent. Cure frequently supersedes improvement as the goal. Few patients are appropriately motivated to tolerate the prolonged discomfort that frequently accompanies recovery.

Hopes are often pinned on new and innovative treatment. A new drug will surely prove superior to an older medication. If it hasn't been tried, then try it; after all, nothing much seems to work anyway.

In our experience, the discarded therapies are often capable of being quite effective. They simply have been abandoned prematurely, or not used confidently and conscientiously. For example, complaining of low back pain and being fifty pounds overweight are irreconcilable conditions. Abusing a powerful analgesic, expecting it to permanently erase a chronic tension headache, leads to rapid drug tolerance and persistent headaches. The mental and physical state of the patient is often a far more significant factor in efficacy than the nature of the treatment. Successful treatment is an active interaction between the patient, doctor, and total program of therapy. A disruption of this triad perpetuates pain and leads to the pain-go-round.

The Pain-Go-Round Explained

The pain-go-round is a symbol. We use it to describe the circular, repetitive process of pain treatment and disappointment, followed by new treatment, new hope, renewed pain, and more disappointment. It characterizes the chronic pain condition. Most chronic pain problems, if left unattended, tend to get worse, not better. Going from one place to another, patients find themselves trapped, searching out additional bits and pieces of information, clues that may help provide a new treatment rationale. Doctors treating these patients find themselves similarly trapped. They may appreciate the extent of a patient's disease; that is, they recognize the severity of the arthritis, the instability of the spine, or the weakness of an intervertebral disk, but find themselves unable to do anything to permanently relieve an individual's suffering.

Doctors and patients find themselves on a merry-go-round, going in circles seeking new and more effective methods of pain control. Through it all, the patient continues to suffer and the physician genuinely tries to provide relief. The original disease, the problem that the medical treatment focuses upon, becomes a minor issue. Pain, the persistent discomfort experienced by the patient, rapidly becomes the central focus of everyone's attention.

What is chronic pain? How do doctors make the diagnosis of chronic pain? The first condition of chronic pain is being ill for longer than four months. While this designation of time may appear arbitrary, it does serve the purpose of differentiating acute from chronic pain. Further, chronic pain is distinguished from the pain of terminal cancer (pain caused by the growth of an untreatable malignant tumor), which is considered to be progressive or intractable pain. The pain of intractable cancer is a direct function of the disease, the result of progressive tumor growth. This is not to imply that some of the techniques for treating chronic pain cannot be ap-

THE
PAIN-GO-ROUND

see lawyer

1 — 3 PM Dr. S
2
3 — cancel lunch w/Jan
4 — 10 AM call Dr. Martin
5
6 — St. Joe's Hosp X-RAY
7
8 — 10 AM neurosurgeon
9
10
11
12 — 2:30 PM Dr. S
13
14 — 1 PM Dr. Long
15
16 — 11 AM Dentist
17
18 — 7 AM St. Joe's Hosp blood tests
19
20 — 10 AM neurosurgeon
21
22
23 — St. Joe's Hosp. tests
24 — cancel dinner w/Jones
25
26
27
28
29 — 9 AM Dr. S
30

P.T.

plied to treating this debilitating pain. They certainly can and in many cases are most useful, but the pain most likely to cause people to board the pain-go-round is generated from benign sources, that is, from nonmalignant sources.

Benign pain is not necessarily a gentle or favorable condition. The quality of being benign refers to the nonmalignant nature of the condition, not to the gentleness of the pain itself. As we have pointed out previously, there are many conditions that can create great misery and suffering.

To understand chronic pain, it's important to consider the medical consequences of living in pain. The Mayo Clinic has worked with a very large number of people who have found themselves *trapped* in chronic pain. These are people caught on the pain-go-round who have found minimal relief from a wide variety of treatments and who ultimately came to the clinic for treatment in the inpatient pain program. The typical patient:

1. Has pain and has had it for a long time (a minimal figure is seven years);
2. Has low back pain (a familiar condition for humans, especially since they stood up on two legs in an exalted expression of mastering their balance by defying the pull of gravity. This pain does not generally stay in the back: it radiates down both legs);
3. Has been hospitalized for a minimum of *six* times for pain-related conditions;
4. Has been operated on at least twice, generally with little, if any, improvement in the pain (not uncommonly, people feel worse—presumably more pain—after surgery);
5. Has pervasively and decisively failed to respond favorably and enthusiastically in any way to any form of conservative medical treatment;
6. Has not worked in two years (for many, the prospect of returning to work is remote: rarely, if ever, is the subject of work mentioned spontaneously; given the extent of the pain, work is irrelevant);
7. Has been receiving compensation payments at sufficient levels to maintain a decent standard of living.

While not all patients with chronic pain fit this profile, these shared characteristics highlight the potential chronic pain holds for destroying a life. People with chronic pain can become absorbed by their pain, live a life regulated by subjective discomfort, and, most unfortunately, not participate in the day-to-day joys of living.

BEFORE YOU JUMP ABOARD THE PAIN-GO-ROUND,
CONSIDER THE FOLLOWING:

Often, what makes chronic pain so difficult to tolerate is the lack of specific reasons for its existence. Pain is not objective; it does not show up on an X ray or appear on your skin, nor can it be measured in the blood. It only hurts, and only the person with pain knows how much it hurts. It is perfectly human to want to see, hear, and touch what you think you feel (and pain, after all, is a perceived feeling). No one wants to live in doubt; if it hurts, it makes perfect sense to find out why. Unfortunately, chronic pain is difficult to chart, measure, and predict. For anyone who suffers with chronic benign pain, the opportunities to become defensive about one's condition are rampant. Before you put your back to the wall and scream, "The pain is not in my head—it's real!" there are several facts about this elusive problem that merit consideration:

1. *Chronic pain is real.* A headache or a backache is a function of strain, which produces actual, physiological, and biochemical changes in your body; however, *it does not mean that something is either broken, torn, or ruptured.*

2. *Chronic benign pain is a natural by-product of many serious but nonfatal progressive diseases.* The most obvious example is arthritis, where inflammation in the bones, ligaments, and joints produces chronic, intermittent pain. Here pain is an inevitable but episodic consequence of disease and cannot be totally eliminated. It can, however, be alleviated. It may not go away forever, but it can be helped.

3. *Certain physical conditions predispose one to experience recurrent bouts of chronic pain.* Aging, loss of muscle tone, obesity, inactivity, poor physical conditioning, even overactivity, may increase the probability of experiencing chronic pain. Clearly, developing good dietary habits, establishing a physical exercise and conditioning program, and learning to regulate stress are key elements in achieving pain control.

4. *Chronic pain is not an all-or-none phenomenon.* It is rare that the pain will completely vanish. It may, but don't bank on it. More likely, a pain condition will vary in intensity over time.

Expecting a condition that has been persistent and nagging to simply go away is unrealistic.

5. *Benign pain is not the "voice" of an isolated injury somewhere in the body; it is an integrated experience, a subjective state having physical, psychological, and emotional input.* The pain conveys a message, it is telling us something about ourselves and the state of our body. Learn to listen critically.

DO ALL PEOPLE WITH PERSISTENT PAIN EVENTUALLY BOARD THE PAIN-GO-ROUND?

Some people learn to conquer their chronic pain and manage to live comfortably. True, some may continue to experience pain, pain that gets better and worse from time to time, but they do not fall apart; they continue to work, enjoy their families, participate in recreation, and fulfill themselves with a variety of interests and activities. They control their pain; they work, love, function, and survive; they do not give up.

There are other individuals who manage, often through no fault of their own, to get caught on the pain-go-round. Once aboard the carrousel they begin to chase the ultimate therapy: the complete pain treatment that will permanently cure their disorder. Insidiously they became prisoners lost in a tumultuous and exhausting search for some medical miracle. Inevitably the structure of their daily lives begins to change. As they become totally absorbed in the attempted management of their pain, getting well becomes a major life task. The chronic pain sufferer quickly becomes a quasi-professional patient as the rigors of treatment replace the routine of daily work and homemaking. Each spin of the pain-go-round brings the sufferer one revolution closer to permanent disability. With each passing month away from the life's established routine, the likelihood of ever getting back to normality rapidly dwindles.

ON THE LIMITS OF SCIENCE—HOW DOCTORS GET CAUGHT ON THE PAIN-GO-ROUND

"Science [and medical science] is built of facts the way a house is built of bricks; but an accumulation of facts is no more science than a pile of bricks is a house."   —HENRI POINCARÉ

As a patient, you should be aware that physicians can get caught up on the pain-go-round as well. An obsessive bunch of people, extremely fearful of "missing something," they leave no stone unturned. And if the pain sufferer goes to more than one doctor, as is often the case, the stones get turned and re-turned a lot of times. As a dedicated professional, the doctor will do almost anything short of touching up an X ray to appease a frustrated patient who demands to know, "What the hell is wrong with me, anyhow?" Faced with a demanding patient who has now failed to respond to the third new "pain medication," the doctor may:

1. Assume he has insufficient evidence and request more expert consultation. This may take the form of specialty referral, where the patient is sent to a neurologist, orthopedic surgeon, psychiatrist, or whatever specialist might presumably shed light on the persistent symptom.

2. Order more complete diagnostic tests or repeat procedures that were either equivocal or negative for hope of uncovering something new.

3. Attempt to "suppress" the pain with a more potent regimen of analgesics. Despite the awareness that most analgesics are short-term measures, persistent complaints from a pain patient make it difficult to refuse any useful help. Saying no is often very difficult.

4. Encourage the patient to persist with the prescribed regimen of conservative treatment, which may include a mild analgesic, muscle relaxant, and some form of activity restriction. By encouraging continuation, the doctor risks creating a sense of futility in the patient. Making some small change is often reassuring. Montaigne commented, "Who ever saw one physician approve of another's prescription, without taking something away or adding something to it?" The same may apply to a doctor's "reconsideration" of his own therapy, especially if the patient complains. (Nonetheless, the premature or hasty abandonment of treatment plans only enhances the patient's insecurity and will escalate the whole process of doubting.)

5. Assume the patient is malingering and does not consciously wish to return to work. Often the physician is correct. Sometimes the pain patient doesn't feel he is "ready." The results of forcing someone to return to work are uniformly disastrous; people can only succeed where they believe they can. Reluctance can easily become a stumbling block—one which the hesitant chronic pain patient usually manages to trip over. Reinjury, almost without exception, puts people back at step one.

6. Choose to dismiss the patient, feeling, perhaps with ample justification, that he has done everything in his power to help and can no longer be of therapeutic benefit.

Doctors are people; well educated and trained, they try to be responsive to the demands of their patients. But when push comes to shove, there is still much that remains unknown, especially about chronic pain. The physician may be subtly lulled aboard the pain-go-round and may try (often despite knowing better) to *cure* a patient's pain. Most often, the doctor wants to be helpful; he wants to be appreciated and may accede to demands that are excessive or slightly unreasonable. Chronic pain is a tough problem, something with which no one wants to live. Often the most difficult task facing the physician is motivating patients to help themselves by being patient and persisting with the current course of treatment.

In our experience, if patients made a greater effort to follow all of their physicians' recommendations (especially the personal recommendations concerning losing weight, maintaining an active exercise program, doing their physical therapy exercises, getting sufficient rest, and all the other assorted information the physician may offer) they would probably find considerable benefits in their treatment. More often than not, the good, solid commonsense "prescriptions" are the most valuable hints in controlling pain. Give your doctor and yourself a chance. Be patient.

A WORD ON HUMAN NATURE, AND CHRONIC PAIN

There may be a growing conviction that Mother Nature moves too slowly. The feeling is not new. Centuries ago Rousseau, the French philosopher, observed, "Nature's instructions are always slow, those of men are generally premature." We are, by breed, impatient.

Conditioned by the media, which harp on the urgency of "quick relief," "immediate satisfaction," and "instantaneous communication," we expect tomorrow to arrive today. In the last national election, the media, through sophisticated computer analysis and telecommunications, predicted President Reagan the winner before the polls closed in California. So rapid was the communication that President Carter conceded before millions of voters could even get to the polls.

Urgency, the need for immediate results, plays an instrumental role in trapping people on the pain-go-round. Certain things can't be rushed, and healing is one. Confucius knew "the desire to have things done quickly prevents their being done thoroughly."

Chronic pain conditions change in a peculiar, though often predictable, manner. Pain improves very slowly, but can get worse precipitously and with alarmingly little provocation.

The rapid rate at which pain accelerates can often be the pain sufferer's downfall, for there is a strong temptation to lose patience during any relapse or acute phase of recovery. Once a chronic pain syndrome is established it will not get better in a day, a week, or even several weeks. Treatment moves slowly, often too slowly to satisfy someone whose capacity to cope is compromised by chronic pain.

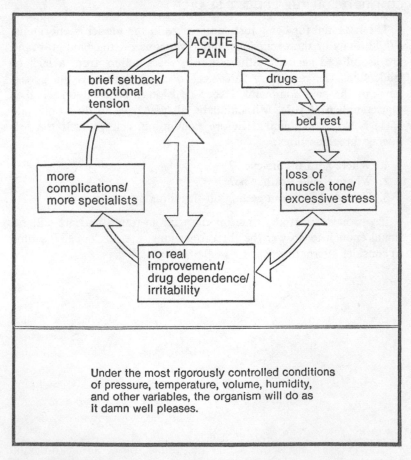

The pain-go-round.

The patient's normal imperturbability begins to weather. Expecting too much from treatments or medications, prematurely returning to full activities, running from doctor to doctor seeking a new or innovative cure, are symptoms of the loss of patience. Eventually all the activity associated with seeking a cure results in mental exhaustion and physical fatigue. The burden on the physician continues to mount. After trying just about everything, the sufferer's patience with innovations dwindles. If something doesn't work fast, then it probably won't work at all. The pain-go-round begins to spin from pain to promise to disappointment.

COMMENTS ON THE ENDLESS SEARCH

The potential for being lost somewhere in the model is enormous. While many of the excursions and diversions on the pain-go-round are useful and necessary, the whole process suffers from a lack of leadership. The regulatory force, the decision maker, is the persistence of the pain complaint. Every decision is based upon whether you complain of pain. Miraculously, all you have to do to end the cycle is stop complaining. Before continuing, ask yourself the following three questions:

1. Where am I on the cycle?
2. Where would I rather be?
3. How do I go about getting off this thing anyway?

If you have spent any time on the pain-go-round and are still rational enough to answer the three questions, there is hope. It's time to consider alternative action.

II

THE CUTTING EDGE OF PAIN: PUTTING THE PIECES BACK TOGETHER

Chapter 5

THE CUTTING EDGE OF PAIN

After three years of recurrent neck pain Laura Silva was exhausted. Fourteen physicians, five physical therapists, and twenty-three medications later, she felt hopeless enough to consent to surgery. The doctors were not very enthusiastic regarding the chance for surgery to relieve her pain, but, convinced that she had no other alternative, Laura wanted to go ahead in the hope that some minimal benefit could be obtained.

The recovery from surgery was extremely slow. She had far more pain after her operation than she had had before. The need for pain-killers became overwhelming. She consumed more narcotic analgesics than she had ever before in her entire life. She developed gastritis, which required extensive treatment and at least two hospitalizations to get it under control. The chronic use of the medications upset her stomach, blurred her thoughts. At times she felt her thinking was so ineffectual that she appeared to be an idiot. Her mood was constantly irritable. Six months after her surgery, her sixteen-year-old daughter left home to go live with Laura's first husband. Although Laura did not dare admit it to anyone, she felt her daughter had done the right thing. Their constant bickering had grown intolerable. Laura could not even stand being with herself.

Despite the best available medical treatment, the spasms in her neck and arms refused to quit. She ingested increasing quantities of narcotics with little effect on her pain. She had quite insidiously developed an enormous tolerance for these once-powerful drugs. Her appetite was so great that she was ashamed to go to the drugstore to fill her prescriptions; she renewed them by phone and had the medication delivered. At one point she discovered she had credit accounts at five different pharmacies.

Then she began getting terrible headaches. They would appear in the morning upon awakening and last throughout the day. It seemed that she always had a headache. A neurological evaluation was normal. A CAT scan was performed which showed no abnormalities. Laura knew why she was getting the headaches. She had become an emotional wreck.

She was overwhelmed. She felt terribly alone and frightened in the world. Not only did her neck hurt but her soul hurt and she did not know where to turn. Quite understandably she felt she had exhausted her resources, that people were tired of hearing about her and her problems. Friends who had once come to visit on a regular basis rarely showed up. When she called and left messages, her messages were unanswered. She wondered where to turn. Someone recommended acupuncture, another person a chiropractor, someone else more surgery. All the uncertainty, the frustration, and the loneliness worsened her pain. She had lost control of her life.

The failure of her marriage, her daughter's decision to live with her father, and now the abuse and dependency on narcotics to relieve her pain were all related to her sore neck. She felt stiff and tense all day. Dreams of actually turning into a skeleton would awaken her during the night with her heart beating and head spinning. Her sleep was so troubled and so violent that she viewed night with alarm and fear. Even the tranquilizers, narcotics, and sleeping pills did not help. She was certain that she would end up in a mental ward. For Laura, there was no relief in sight, just endless torment. To go to a hospital was both her greatest fear and her secret wish, for then at last the long waiting would be ended. She could at last admit defeat.

There are millions of people who, like Laura Silva, spend endless nights tossing and turning, pacing through a house where everyone else is peacefully resting. There are those who take meals alone or rush from the dinner table for fear of sitting up too long. There are many who would be working but know that any excessive exertion could flare their problem, perhaps sending them back home for a week or a month or perhaps for good. Such is the course of chronic pain.

In your mind's eye, visualize a tranquil, secluded pond. A peaceful scene filled with lilies, some fish, perhaps a frog or two. Someone comes along and casts a stone into the pond; it creates a splash, an initial disturbance. Then waves, ripples of turbulence, radiate out from the splash, washing to the shore in all directions. Imagine throwing stone after stone into the water repeatedly, day after day. Not only would the surface of the pool be in a constant state of agitation, but the entire equilibrium of the pond would be drastically changed. The fish would die off, the frogs would leave, even the water lilies would have trouble surviving. Living in pain is similar to life in the disturbed pond. The forces that normally create a harmonious and balanced environment are disturbed. Things change: as pain persists, the balance is disturbed.

When we speak of a chronic pain syndrome, we address the total effects of living in pain. We strongly believe that pain disturbs all aspects of a person's life. Chronic pain is a disease whose symptoms may include the development of stress-related illness; the stress of constant worry may aggravate an ulcer or precipitate a bout of alcoholism in a vulnerable individual. Pain changes the personality, erodes self-esteem and confidence, strains the bonds of family relations, and depresses the mood. Just as the life in the pond is eventually unbalanced by the damage of the stones, the stress of living in pain overwhelms the individual in his environment.

The following chapters explore the dynamic effects of chronic pain and offer some practical suggestions for handling these problems.

Chapter 6

COPING WITH THE STRESS OF PAIN

The Stress Me Generation

They were spawned in the postwar years to enjoy the best of American life, complete with modern kitchen appliances, two-car garages, and the privilege of enjoying rock-and-roll music. This new, socially conscious generation gained national prominence camouflaged as Yippies, hippies, and the SDS. They seized the conscience of social awareness and forced it down American throats.

As students, they yearned for individuality but came out looking remarkably similar in dress and appearance. They maintained focus and gained momentum and credibility by popularizing resistance to a war of attrition in the stinking swamps of Asia. They were to become the "Me Generation." They were appalled by apathy and resented the government. Their defiance overflowed; they denounced the narrow material pursuits of their parents and pedantic conventions of capitalistic vocations, choosing actively to drop out, sit in, or just get high. They mauled the previously unmolested social boundaries. Good taste waned; no taste prevailed.

For much of the sixties and into the seventies, the Me Generation stuffed itself into tight jeans, smoked a lot of pot, drank some Pepsi, eventually became "Peppers," and in the process raised the general level of social consciousness. With it they brought the national anxiety quotient (NAQ) to a new high.

This generation made stress a household word in America. The compliant acceptance of dogmatic bureaucracy that characterized the postwar era ended as Americans began to take notice of the stress that was encroaching upon their electronic lives. Those incidental little pressures, such as the endless hordes of cars, environmental pollution, escalating inflation, even the expectation of nuclear contamination, have become woven into the fabric of people's daily lives. More than minor annoyances, these stresses are now seen as incessant additive ingredients in the creation of physical and emotional illnesses. Life in America echoes the conditions of stress, and people have begun to recognize its incredibly deleterious effect on their good health and longevity.

To those of us whose hearts palpitate with each turn of the page of the morning paper, the experience of stress may be at least in part a criterion of sanity. Being sensitive to the dangers that surround us, we are bound to secrete and hypersecrete all the hormones that alert our bodies to potential danger. Yet stress is not universal. Not every one of us experiences this "alerting" response to our environment. Further, stress does not cause disease and illness uniformly in response to changes in the environment. The striking truth is that the experience and effects of stress are highly individual and variable. Moreover, some individuals exist who seemingly thrive on stress, actually becoming healthier and more effective in its presence. Other people crumble, developing stress-related illness and emotional disorders, and experiencing a gross disruption in functioning.

Stress can best be understood as having two components: an external condition, or the social, professional, and family environment a person lives in, and an internal condition—the mental, emotional, and physical condition of the individual himself.

It is generally agreed that certain jobs or conditions are highly stressful. For example, air traffic controllers are at high risk to develop stress-related illness (peptic ulcer, hypertension, cardiac disease) presumably because the external conditions of their job are stressful enough to promote excessive internal stress. By studying air traffic controllers, scientists have been able to distinguish the particular environmental conditions that are stressful to the degree that they can create mental and physical disease. While these conditions do not always create disease, stress-related diseases may occur and be aggravated in an environment where:

1. The potential for personal failure is high.
2. Multiple simultaneous demands are placed on the individual.
3. Great expectations predominate.
4. Multiple centers compete for a single individual's attention.
5. There is minimal time for momentary mental unwinding and revitalization.
6. Self-absorption and personal isolation are regular features.

7. The potential danger posed by inadvertent distractions is high.
8. Personal efforts are compromised by a sense of helplessness or impotence.

While these are not the only conditions of stress, they are certainly environmental factors that affect air traffic controllers and make their work and their life remarkably stressful. But these conditions can affect anyone, in any place, in any job.

As potentially stressful as the air traffic controllers' environment may be, not every controller develops a stress-related illness. Nor does each controller develop the same disease. Individuals show great variation in the capacity to handle stress; that is, to function under high-pressure conditions without becoming mentally or physically ill.

Researchers have reproduced many "psychosomatic" human illnesses by subjecting animals to various conditions of stress. No one will say that stress is the sole or even the pivotal factor in the creation of a major illness. However, it is widely accepted that excessive stress is a significant influence in the development of many major diseases.

A heightened awareness of the brain's regulatory potential in health and disease is emerging from research in neuroendocrine studies. The brain, of course, is the nerve center of the body, where information collected in all the areas of the body is processed. As the brain processes input, it communicates with tissues and organs by sending nerve impulses through the spine and out through peripheral nerves to tissues, organs, and muscles. These messages may be commands for voluntary motion (walking, talking, etc.) or involuntary activity (breathing, heartbeat). But nerve impulses are only one means of communication. The release of neurohormones is another very active means by which the brain communicates with the body. Neurohormones are chemical messengers that communicate the brain's commands to various tissues and organs. For example, the neurohormone *vasopressin,* which is produced in the brain in response to perceived danger or stress, is released into the circulation and effects changes in the kidneys that help adapt the body to potential danger. Specifically, vasopressin forces the kidney to conserve fluid (antidiuretic effect) as a prerequisite to raising the blood pressure.

Scientists are just now beginning to appreciate the complex and elaborate neurohormonal connections that link the brain to virtually every tissue and organ in the body. The term psychosomatic means that mind as well as body plays a role in the creation of disease. Whereas it was once thought that 50 to 70 percent of disease was psychosomatic in origin, it is now felt by some experts that upwards of 95 percent of all illness is psychosomatic in nature.

MODIFYING STRESS

In 1908, Drs. Robert Yerkes and John Dodson of Harvard University Medical School first described the potentially beneficial and ultimately deleterious effects of stress on human performance and efficiency. They demonstrated that as stress increased, so did efficiency and productivity. As human systems, we depend on a certain amount of stress to motivate us to function effectively.

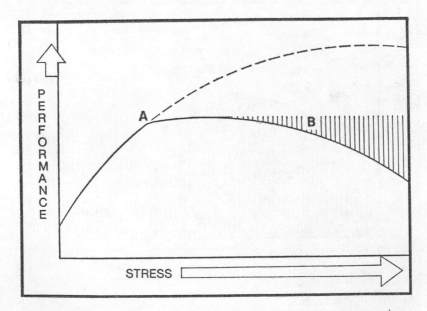

Yerkes-Dodson curve. Dotted curve represents untapped coping potential. Shaded area represents lost performance.

Up to a point (A), stress enhances performance. At point A, stress is maximally tolerated, creating conditions of maximum performance and efficiency. As stress continues to increase, efficiency and performance begin to fall off. At point B the level of stress exceeds the capacity to cope; performance falls off and the organism begins to experience excessive stress. (See crosshatched area.) This curve shows how a person increases his capacity to handle increasingly high levels of stress until an optimum point is reached. But what happens to the person with chronic pain? Does he maintain the same capacity to cope with stress?

In the figure below we have diagrammed the effect of chronic pain on the Yerkes-Dodson model. The presence of pain significantly changes the configuration of the curve. The persistence of pain creates a "dead-weight effect" on the Yerkes-Dodson curve, dragging down the slope of the coping potential. Chronic pain syndromes distort the organism's ability to handle stress, because the stress of coping with pain reduces the strength available to manage environmental stress.

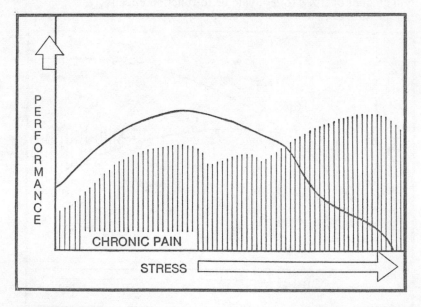

The drain of chronic pain.

The following stress test is designed to help you evaluate the level of your coping capacity. If you doubt the validity of the albatross effect of chronic pain on the Yerkes-Dodson coping curve, simply take the stress test and carefully consider the results.

How Stressful Is My Pain?

Answer Key

1 frequently
2 occasionally
3 hardly ever

1. _____ Pain causes me to leave the table before others are finished eating.
2. _____ Pain makes me irritable.
3. _____ When I wake up in the morning I dread the start of a new day.
4. _____ I am likely to lose patience with problems that can't be easily solved.
5. _____ I find it hard to be objective and realistic.
6. _____ Drinking alcohol makes my pain less burdensome.
7. _____ I fail to get any exercise during the course of the day.
8. _____ Entertaining friends increases my pain discomfort.
9. _____ When I visit the doctor, pain is my usual complaint.
10. _____ I use narcotic pain relievers.
11. _____ Sexual relations are difficult and tense.
12. _____ When I am hurting I want to be left alone.
13. _____ My children find me grouchy.
14. _____ Friends avoid asking me about my pain.
15. _____ I take more than ten pills a day.
16. _____ I have sexual relations less than once a week.
17. _____ I frequently call in sick to my job.
18. _____ Life's problems seem to pile up.
19. _____ I will leave a movie or show early because of physical discomfort.
20. _____ I have the feeling that my husband/wife is not as close to me as he/she once was.

SCORE   Less than 30—Major stress
             30–45—Moderate stress
         More than 45—Little effect

We have found that most people with chronic pain will record scores below 42, indicating a moderate to severe stress reaction caused by long-standing pain.

Because the consequences of pain plus stress can be so devastating, some simple steps to help reduce the stress of anxiety are given below. Persons with scores below 42 *must* try to master these hints. The alternative is a life plagued by the very stresses that shorten life. Persons with scores above 42 should also find that following this advice will have beneficial effects.

- When you find yourself losing patience, *stop*. Just the pause will break the anxiety-to-irritability cycle. Try to identify the cause of your irritability. Be specific. Do not take your pain out on those around you. Isolation will soon follow.
- After you have identified the stressor, always take an active stance in changing it. The act of confronting an appropriate irritant implies that you may control it; control reduces anxiety, which in turn reduces irritability and pain.
- Always plan one enjoyable or interesting activity for the next day. Write it down and plan it out the night before. It gives you something to look forward to when everything else may appear bleak.
- Explain to your family or friends that you may have to interrupt a dinner or a meeting to get up and walk around. They will understand even if you think they will not. Very often people are afraid that others will not understand, so they don't even ask.
- Always break up your tasks into small parts. People with nagging pain become overwhelmed easily. Keep from becoming overwhelmed and you will keep from becoming irritable. See Chapter 19 for some helpful hints.
- Always practice the relaxation exercises given in Chapter 15—not sometimes, but every day. Studies confirm that even a fifteen-minute break twice a day can mean the difference between stress and relief.
- Let out some tension with ten to twenty minutes of physical exercise (to tolerance) per day. It is worth repeating that this lets out a great deal of tension in a healthy way.
- Reducing your dependence on narcotics will reduce your mood swings. See Chapter 13 ("Medicines for Pain").
- See your friends and engage in your normal activities as much as possible. You will, within certain limits, have your pain whether or not you talk with your neighbor or sit at a bench

doing the woodworking project you like. Just exercise good judgment.

■ Save a treat for the end of the day—a hot bath, or some ice cream, or a piece of music. It allows you to look forward to the end of the day with some brightness.

JUST HOW STRESSFUL IS PAIN?

Pain is a most unique stress. It is a stress because it causes an alteration in the way we function. Chronic pain, because you always have it, will change the way you do everything. Stress sits like an umbrella over the pain system, incessantly pressuring, coaxing, and taunting you to respond. "How long can I tolerate this party before I lose my patience and have to go lie down?" or "If this headache doesn't go away I'm going to scream" or "My back is so stiff after walking I'm going to stop going out!"

Pain creates stress by:

1. Its pervasive, nagging quality, creating a constant state of physical discomfort.
2. Limiting your capacity to cope not only with the pain but with the functions and responsibility of daily life. The constant pressure of coping with pain reduces the time and energy for handling all of life's other problems. This is why people with chronic pain are more likely to develop problems with jobs, family, friends, etc. They have less energy and problem-solving time to devote to other areas.
3. Creating fear. It plagues us with fear of the unknown, the uncertain. "What is wrong with me?" "Do I have cancer?" "If I do what the doctors tell me, why isn't the problem going away?"
4. Stealing away your time. Pain perpetuates procrastination. Often problems that could be easily solved accumulate under the stress of chronic pain, creating an illusion of constant crisis. Time spent in pain, worried about how to handle pain, is lost time.
5. Compromising your ability to function in the activities of daily living. The patient with chronic pain loses his physical and mental effectiveness. The normal responsibilities and pleasures of daily living become a burden. Being unable to work at your

own occupation, feeling the need to periodically stop what you're doing to rest, experiencing discomfort during sexual activity, are all potentially threatening situations.

Chronic pain is the great uncoper. It undoes the job of putting your life together. By reducing your problem-solving ability, it makes easy jobs tough and difficult problems impossible. Before long everyone begins to bend a little. The uncoper takes over and any one or more of the following personality changes may occur:

1. GENERALIZED FUSE SHORTENING (GFS)

This may also be known as the explosive or unpredictable personality. In healthy individuals a residual amount of energy exists to cope with the broad variety of generalized stresses. People who are generally healthy can absorb a lot of abuse before losing patience. Chronic pain is especially notorious for draining away the residual coping buffer. The sufferer feels he has more than he can handle with his pain. Any trauma will burst the bubble.

Identifying the syndrome can be easy. The afflicted individual is generally prone to bouts of yelling, screaming, or crying. Generally, the precipitating event is trivial.

Coworkers, family members, and friends are easily recognizable. They develop the *eggshell syndrome*—fear of saying or doing anything that might provoke the pain sufferer. Never quite certain what might or might not be offensive, they approach every confrontation with extreme caution, as if walking on eggs. People at work request transfer to another department, go out of their way to avoid an office or desk, and make absolutely certain that if they have anything to say to you they catch you in a good mood. At home your children immediately stop talking, straighten up, and appear miraculously innocent when you walk into the room. They leave the table early, spend much of their free time outside, and rarely have friends visit.

2. BIG DEALISM

Another fairly common response to the stress of chronic pain is finding 101 reasons why something, anything, is a big deal. It really doesn't matter how insignificant the event, the big dealer can give a masterfully foolproof explanation of why he can't do it. As there is always an element of truth in all but the most ill-conceived or frivolous arguments, the big dealer always has a logical starting point. "Walking tires me out, makes my back ache," "If I don't lie down during the day the pain becomes unbearable," and "How do you expect me to lose weight—I barely eat one meal a day as it is," are but a sampling of common big dealisms.

The manifestations of big dealism are fairly obvious. Generally, the family of the pain patient gradually shoulders the responsibilities of the big dealer. Tasks are willingly taken over by zealous helpers. In time, the big dealer finds he has fewer genuinely difficult, time-consuming, or tedious tasks for which he is responsible and about which he can legitimately complain. Forced to continue big dealing, the pain sufferer descends the hierarchy, finding new and previously simple tasks to convert from molehills to mountains.

Stress has the capacity to make every usual and common activity a burden. But why are pain sufferers so likely to be trapped in this sea of helplessness?

Many pain sufferers are ashamed of their condition. It is quite common for patients to comment that they are no longer entertaining guests, accepting social invitations, or even going out to a movie. They feel constantly fatigued and drained of initiative. Consequently they do less and less. Often, having suffered for months with a persistent pain problem, people get worn out just explaining the stagnant situation to their friends.

Frank Belman, a foreman in a large steel mill, was incapacitated by chronic cervical (neck) pain. He is the perfect example of big dealism in action.

Once able to help out on the line, forge, and lift large iron castings, he was incapacitated after severely twisting his shoulder in a bad spill. Frank was the original macho man. Before his injury he never complained or allowed any task to overwhelm him. He could not imagine going back to his job until he was fully able to do *every* physical task he had done prior to his injury. For him doing less meant losing the respect of his men. Further, he didn't want anyone from work to visit him during his recovery. He wasn't up to having people see him in his present state. "What good am I? The people at work were nice enough to inquire when I got hurt, but do they really care? They're not interested unless I can do the job they hired me for." He was ashamed of being sick, could not accept feeling less virile and able, and would do nothing constructive to help himself unless he was totally better.

Gradually Frank's shame spilled over to his relations with family and neighbors. Frank, always the superb host, refused company unless he could serve them to perfection. "If someone needs a drink I feel obliged to get up and fill their glass. Preparing a gourmet dinner —*al dente*—has always been routine protocol. I just can't bring myself to not be a good host and right now everything is a big deal."

Over a period of several months Frank stopped driving, shopping for groceries, running routine errands, even eating his meals with the family. He could not tolerate doing any physical activity below his former level of efficiency, but the amount of effort required to do so became enormous.

In addition to losing friends and becoming a social outcast, his motivation to get well evaporated. The emptiness of his social and personal life stripped his confidence. Not handling routine responsibilities, he became fearful of his ability to do anything. From his perspective everything was a big deal.

3. THE CRISIS MAKERS

Those who knew Andrea Marsh never knew quite what to expect from her. She was unpredictable. Although she was only thirty-nine years old, a bad case of arthritis had severely debilitated her left hip. The constant pain was a physical handicap that kept her from performing routine functions and from standing for any prolonged period. Ed, her ever willing husband, worked double time to try to take up the slack.

Like clockwork, every few weeks her arthritis would flare up and send her to bed for several days. Andrea hated these interruptions in her daily schedule. She was an active person who relished overextending herself. Being indisposed several days a month enticed her to overschedule her "up days." No project was too complex or time-consuming for Andrea. In addition to caring for her three children ages five to eleven, she was a Cub Scout den mother, PTA chairperson, and free-lanced as an amateur potter at the local craft shows. While mere mortals would find her schedule exhausting, Andrea thrived. She flourished in the frantic pace.

Arthritis came as a shock. Never having been ill before in her life, she felt the idea of paying special attention to her health was repugnant. She was unequivocally opposed to incorporating any time to relax in her schedule. Eventually, the condition advanced to an unbearable state. Left with no alternative, Andrea retired to bed to rest her hip. Several days in bed generally rejuvenated her sufficiently to be able to carry on her full gamut of family and community responsibilities. She was the ultimate trouper.

At first glance, Andrea appeared to be a whirlwind of activity. Closer scrutiny revealed flaws.

Cub Scout meetings regularly degenerated into cupcake-tossing contests. Project materials were never ordered in sufficient supply. Imagine having twelve eleven-year-olds intent on making twelve pairs of moccasins from only six pairs of soles. The day's outing to the county fair, planned months in advance, was marred because Andrea failed to call the bus company for transportation. The rains came, leaving a dozen waterlogged cub scouts wading in puddles waiting for the unsummoned buses.

Andrea Marsh's arthritis caused her enough pain to slow the pace of her life. Unfortunately, Andrea's mind didn't slow down. The tempo of her drives and plans continued to exceed her ability to get things done. In addition to a pain problem, she developed a stress problem.

Since she was never quite able to catch up and finish everything she started, her family and friends all too frequently found themselves mopping up. Genuinely repentant, she doled out apologies profusely. It didn't matter, everyone around her was tired of cleaning up her mess.

Worst of all, the stress and tension of her life increased her pain. Gradually her "down time" increased. More unannounced absences, more days in bed. Discouragement with lack of progress prompted her to make premature and often inappropriate decisions about her treatment. She switched orthopedic surgeons, but whenever she found a new physician, she failed to benefit because she couldn't listen. Her strong need to be well and the stress of pain fueled her impatience. She just couldn't wait.

THE LARGER QUESTIONS

In relating these case histories, we want to highlight the intricate relationship between physical pain and stress.

Severe pain quickly becomes the most important issue in someone's life. People will reorganize their lives and regulate their behavior to compensate for the extra pressures created by physical pain. It becomes the number one mental concern.

Almost every patient with chronic pain will show evidence of marked concern, in spite of rigorous, although often subtle efforts, to minimize such concern. The potential questions are so stressful that they require minimization.

The immediate problem for the acute patient is: "If I hurt this much, there must be something terribly wrong." Pain goes with injury as bread goes with butter. It's a natural. Convincing someone in persistent pain that there is no physical injury or disease is nearly impossible. Justifiably, no one wants to believe the pain is "imagined." If you feel it in your body it must be in your body. It is contrary to human nature to experience pain without trying to place it. Unplaced, free-floating pain is far more stressful than pain that has an origin.

Once the pain is placed somewhere in the body, the question "How long will I have to suffer this way?" becomes a major issue. The persistence of pain, despite very aggressive and conscientious treatment, can create incredible stress. Because things don't get better quickly and recovery is plagued with frequent setbacks, there is a tendency to exaggerate the possibility of lasting or permanent damage.

While these concerns are rarely articulated, they are commonly the source of severe stress in patients with chronic pain. They cause stress in people because to some extent they are unanswerable questions. Hashing them over time and again doesn't clarify the issue. A lot of mental energy is wasted that could otherwise be spent learning to cope.

ON COPING: A DIGRESSION ON CALCULATORS, CHILDREN, AND COMMITMENT

We fear that the current generation of children nurtured with the aid of pocket calculators may become adults who can't multiply. Multiplication has always held a certain fascination for us. There is a genuine sense of assurance in figuring up the price of a dozen apples at eight cents (or thirty cents) apiece, or knowing how many miles you get on ten gallons of gas. It's interesting that when people's memories begin to fade, one of the last functions they lose is the ability to multiply. Having numbers ingrained so deeply and using them fairly frequently serves a purpose.

Things are different today. Pocket calculators in a variety of shapes and sizes, with names like Little Professor and Mr. Wizard, are rampant. Kids use them to do their homework. The manufacturers virtually give them away. It's a bit like hooking someone on drugs. The addictive potential is immense. Hook the kid early, create an electronic dependence, and by the time he gets to the fifth grade you are guaranteed a lifetime customer.

It's Satlinger's Law that states, "It works better if you plug it in— unless of course it runs on batteries." Most electronic devices do run on batteries, and their portability makes them virtually indispensable.

It is not unusual for us to meet an individual who has successfully avoided human contact with the aid of electronic devices. A patient of ours had become an expert at chess without ever playing another person; he did it all with a computer. Years ago, he would have been forced to join the chess club, deal with the social anxiety of talking to other kids, and somehow work out a place for himself. Now he keys an electronic chessmate, stays harbored in the refuge of his own room for five years, and emerges as a chess expert without ever having to speak to another person.

The problem with all these electronic conveniences is that they help people avoid themselves. In the nineteen-eighties a growing majority of Americans are resisting the necessity of coping. The conveniences of modern living have created an aura of helplessness that is insidiously but progressively engulfing our collective consciousness. Coping has come to mean resignation. We have come to delegate the responsibility for ourselves to *things,* such as calculators and computers. The challenge of self-directed achievement, the ability to master our own fate, has been minimized by the advent of electronic wizardry. In *The Sane Society,* the noted psychoanalyst Erich Fromm warned, "The danger of the past was that men became slaves, the danger of the future is that men may become robots."

A new generation of jobs has evolved that specializes in coping with problems for other people—anything to improve the standard of living. People are paid to sit in helicopters and watch traffic conditions, lest we get stuck in a bottleneck on the way home. Child psychologists spawn paperbacks galore divulging the ultimate secrets of coping with infants, toddlers, and, of course, adolescents. Even the economists saturate the media with advice on coping with the upcoming financial crisis. The world is filled with self-styled experts who liberally bestow their solutions on a rapidly enlarging consumer market.

Genuine persistence and the stick-to-itiveness of the self-determined are rapidly evaporating qualities of the American personality.

The lure of easy solutions, shifting responsibility, and diminished personal input in a society where technological progress outstrips the human capacity to keep pace has eroded the confidence of many who are coaxed to ignore the challenges of self-doubt. How much confidence can you have to survive the stress of day-to-day living if you haven't even learned to multiply?

Our institutions have lost their stabilizing potential. The nuclear family, once the stronghold of traditional values, now sits mesmerized by television. Electronic games such as Atari and Startrack also allow us to choose distraction over introspection. As a culture, we battle the temptation to avoid tension and conflict. Comfort and self-indulgence are omnipresent dangers threatening the capacity to learn about ourselves and the ones we love.

Nothing is sacred. There are localities in the United States where there are more divorces than marriages. Logically, that is not a trend that could continue for very long. If your relationship gets stale, get out, start anew, play it over again. While 50 percent of first marriages end in divorce, 60 percent of second marriages finish with a split.

AND WHAT DOES ALL THIS HAVE TO DO WITH PAIN?

Perhaps you wonder what multiplying, computer games, calculators, and divorce have to do with chronic pain.

Coping—a critical human process in controlling chronic pain—has been severely impaired by a media-led, sociologically instigated assault on self-determination. Simply stated, we have learned to give up too easily. In the battle to control chronic pain, the premature termination of appropriate treatment is the single greatest cause of persistent difficulty. Coping with pain requires using all of your internal resources, the full range of mental and physical faculties. Coping means creating a positive outcome out of even the most outrageous or adverse conditions. Washington Irving commented, "Some minds seem almost to create themselves, spring up under every disadvantage and working their solitary but irresistible way through a thousand obstacles."

All too often, the chronic pain sufferer delegates the responsibility to some physician or therapist ordained to eradicate pain. Coping with pain connotes a state of forbearance—an immutable condition. The pain sufferer rapidly assumes the cloak of helpless victim awaiting deliverance. Only the end never comes. While it's good to hope, the waiting can spoil it. Pain becomes a static situation and the victim is hopelessly imprisoned in the jail of his body.

You've Got to Want *to Do It*

What is coping? How does someone mentally cope with a physical problem like chronic pain?

Some time ago we received a call from a prospective patient inquiring about our pain control program. She wanted to know what treatments we offered, whether medication was used, and specifically how we planned to "treat" her pain. We summarized our program as one which helped people manage and cope with the problems of chronic pain, at which point the woman informed me she knew how to *cope;* what she was interested in was getting rid of her pain. She was not interested in coping better: she wanted to *be* better!

Does it sound familiar? It should. Many people feel this way.

In the face of chronic pain you can and probably should look in two directions: externally, to the world of medical science, for the latest, most effective treatments and specialists, and internally, to the mental and physical resources you already possess. This inner search for your innate skills, talents, courage, and strength is coping. Don't sell it short.

"People see or read about persons—not just yogis—whose minds can cope with pain or can control bleeding, and there is a gee-whiz reaction akin to what happens when people see bears ride bicycles or when they see a woman sawed in half at the circus. Yet nothing in the field of vended magic is as arresting as new knowledge about the regulatory possibilities of mind. A new frontier in the understanding of life is being opened up. It represents one of the main challenges confronting medical science today."

The quotation from Norman Cousins, who for forty or so years has been editor of the *Saturday Review,* critic, philosopher, and spokesman for international cooperation, is taken from an article he wrote on learning to control his pain. When doctors attending him all but gave up, he decided to take events into his own hands.

Cousins discovered within himself the power of positive emotions and their enormous potential for healing. For years, medical science has shown the ill effects of negative emotions: how such emotions as fear, rage, frustration, and anger produce hormonal, biochemical, and ultimately physical changes in the human body. Increased blood pressure, blood-vessel constriction, excess adrenal secretion, over-stimulation of gastric acid, and muscle spasm are all changes that can be uniformly produced by the acute and chronic effects of negative emotions. The so-called stress illnesses have recently become an important focus of medical research.

Coping is the key to reversing the adverse effects of excessive stress. Chronic pain produces constant stress; channeling the stress into positive adaptive mechanisms is sign of a healthy individual.

TO LIVE A LONG AND HEALTHY LIFE

There is a growing volume of evidence that the people who cope with the stresses of life most successfully, those who achieve fame, wealth and success, are also the most healthy. In 1976 the Metropolitan Life Insurance Company conducted a study of the top three executives of each of the Fortune 500 Companies comparing them to a matched sample of men (people of the same age, race and sex, but not of equal socioeconomic status). They found that the corporate executives had a third less morbidity (serious illness) than the sample population. Contrary to the plush, easy life-style that might be expected, these executives worked rigorous schedules, as much as six days a week, twelve or more hours a day. They handled enormous pressures on a regular basis and as a group managed to maintain active close family relationships. Remarkably, they accomplished all this without getting sick, or at least not as much as those who worked less effectively.

George Vaillant, a psychiatrist at the Harvard University School of Medicine, has conducted a longitudinal study of a group of men over the course of their lives. The study started in the nineteen-forties. Several hundred freshmen at a famous liberal eastern university (presumably Harvard) were randomly selected as a study sample. Each was studied, interviewed, and questioned with the goal of assessing their individual coping capacities. Two questions arose: Were coping patterns identifiable? If they were, could they be predictors of future health status? Each study member was followed with a battery of interviews and questionnaires over the course of the next forty years.

The results of this study were complex and detailed. However, it was noted that numerous psychological factors correlated with the development of problems in later life (including alcoholism, drug abuse, divorce and other personal problems, and the development of physical diseases). The people who coped well in college continued to cope well as adults. They developed fewer serious illnesses, had better, more stable family lives, felt happier and more satisfied with themselves. They had come to terms with their lives and their internal and external environments; they simply adapted better.

We believe that people can be taught to cope and, as a result, learn to prevent the development and halt the progression of disease. Unfortunately, we may be beginning the whole process all too late in life. It would be advantageous to educate our children not only in academic subjects but also the techniques of coping and life adaptation. Nonetheless, perhaps the place to begin is with ourselves.

To a person with chronic pain, the idea of prevention may seem a bit irrelevant. You may think that, after all, you already *have* the disease. But chronic pain syndromes are not static. They vacillate, getting better and worse over time. They are constantly changing in response to a multitude of internal and external stimuli. Identifying these stimuli and controlling their dynamic forces is a major step on the road to recovery. From day to day you will have the opportunity to function or not to function. The choice, in large measure, is yours.

Some Suggestions for Coping with Chronic Pain

Jean-Paul Sartre, the French philosopher and writer, established his existential belief around the principle that man was nothing much other than what he made of himself. Living with chronic pain puts you at a distinct disadvantage. The stress of constant pain, concomitant depression, and the other associated discomforts can compromise even the best coping skills. The following list of coping principles is neither complete nor definitive, but it is hoped that it will be provocative and stimulate some reassessment.

PRINCIPLE ONE: Never Take Life Too Seriously
Life is hard enough. Add to that the burden of being sick, out of work, or unable to participate in the joy and recreation of pleasurable diversion and you have a sorry state of affairs.

We are not suggesting that you ignore your health or behave frivolously and irresponsibly, just that you add enough blurring to your vision to avoid some of the more stark realities. Seeing things clearly and concisely is not always an advantage. The real world is not easy to live in. As we age, our bodies begin to wear out. Meeting every adversity and setback with grim sobriety can be grueling. Staying sober is fine, but not all the time.

The burden of chronic pain is not light. A well-developed sense of humor, a veneer to coat over your frustration, and a bit of good old human denial can help soften the blow of certain "hard realities."

PRINCIPLE TWO: Accept a Certain Amount of Uncertainty

No one is perfect. Just because you visit a doctor, go through the clinical examination and a series of laboratory tests and X rays, and pay a fee, don't expect a complete description of your disease, how you got it, why you hurt, and when you'll be well again. At best, medicine is an art and doctors are practitioners. We are still refining the art.

Marcel Proust elegantly summarized the situation: "Medicine being a compendium of the successive and contradictory mistakes of medical practitioners, when we summon the wisest of them to our aid, the chances are we may be relying on a scientific truth the error of which will be recognized in a few years' time." Truth can be very relative.

Tolerating a modicum of uncertainty from your physician as well as yourself will not only prevent some major disappointment, but may actually improve the quality of care you receive. Knowing "everything," always having an immediate solution, is more likely a defense or an avoidance of the real problem than a measure of the doctor's expertise. Uncertainty can be a great teacher, especially when it forces you and your doctor to look longer, search more critically, and wait a bit more patiently before thinking you really understand.

PRINCIPLE THREE: Avoid Spending Too Much Time with Yourself

Your own good company, no matter how engaging and stimulating, can wear thin if not mixed from time to time with the best and worst of friends. Variety, while not necessarily the spice of life, helps provide an appetizing mix.

"The person who tries to live alone will not succeed as a human being. His heart withers if it does not answer another heart. His mind shrinks away if he hears only the echoes of his own thoughts and finds no other inspiration." These reflections on the dangers of solitude are from Pearl Buck's writings. They apply unconditionally to the person with pain who feels a tendency to run away and hide, avoiding the well-meaning but "burdensome" intrusion of friends and relatives.

But the real danger of seclusion is not the avoidance of people; it is the indulgence of self. Too much introspection and self-analysis can distort perspectives and make you all too aware of your pain. Oliver Wendell Holmes had the good sense to observe, "If you mean to keep as well as possible, the less you think about your health the better." A little self-knowledge, especially in the wrong hands, is a dangerous thing.

PRINCIPLE FOUR: Learn To Lean on People—Not a Lot, but Just Enough to Let Them Know You're There

Independence is a fine thing, but being dependent is sometimes better. Every healthy adolescent who ever felt his oats spent the better part of his teenage years figuring out ways to escape the stupidity, indulgence, and "old-fashioned mentality" of his family, especially his parents—only to discover, as he navigated the portals of adulthood, that people like his family were pretty good to have around. Learning how to love people, be able to depend on them, and not suffocate them in the process is no small feat. It's actually a lot harder to learn the rules of dependency than to deny the need for people.

"Every man expects somebody or something to help him," says Edgar Howe in *Ventures in Common Sense*. Despite its apparent simplicity, the lesson is often denied. All too often, the person in pain takes the stoic but foolish position that he has already been too much of a burden and now must *do it himself*. This struggle for independence occurs at a time when one might reasonably and appropriately request help and advice.

Knowing when to ask for help, feeling comfortable allowing another person to care for you without shame, guilt, or self-recrimination, is a sign of maturity and often a major lever in helping to avoid real pain.

PRINCIPLE FIVE: Don't Think About Things, Do Them

"He who would make serious use of his life must act as though he had a long time to live and must schedule his time as though he were about to die" (Emile Littré).

It seems that if you have enough time to sit around and think about things, you'll come up with a slew of reasons why they can't possibly be done. Time is a valuable commodity. It can be used wisely, hardly used, or simply wasted.

One trap of being chronically ill is loss of structure. Much can be said about the ill effects of stress and the pressure of daily living, but having a schedule, a place to go in the morning where they expect you to show up and be on time and do your job, goes a long way in preventing mental illness. It's nice to know that no matter how much you hate your job, despise your boss, or dislike the guy who sits behind you, when push comes to shove you can at least complain about it. Spending a lot of time pondering the course of your life, the destiny of the stars, even the likelihood of nuclear holocaust, is the kind of excessive rumination that leads to a bad case of depression.

Whatever you can do to get something done, do it. When pain sufferers develop a false sense of pride, relatively small accomplishments can wane in the light of previous life achievements. Many very important people have been disabled with chronic pain just because they couldn't allow themselves the embarrassment of stepping down a rung or two. No less an authority than Sir Arthur Conan Doyle, creator of the inscrutable Sherlock Holmes, observed —or, rather, had Holmes observe—"It has long been an axiom of mine that the little things are infinitely more important." Let yesterday pass, do what you can today, and get on with it.

PRINCIPLE SIX: Keep It Simple

"To be simple is the best thing in the world; to be modest is the next best thing. I am not so sure about being quiet." G. K. CHESTERTON

PRINCIPLE SEVEN: When in Doubt, Do What You Think Is Best

There are good decisions and bad decisions, and in the course of a lifetime you have ample opportunity to make a fair share of each. Predictably, someone will always have a better solution to your problems than the one you're using. After all, if your solution was so good how come you're still in pain? With that kind of sound rhetorical logic it's pretty hard to resist the temptation to abandon ship. Indecision, uncertainty, even failures, are part of the recovery process. The greatest failure, however, is the mistake you let someone make for you. Follow-the-leader is fine for teaching compliance in elementary school, but if you have a pain problem it will win you a permanent seat on the pain-go-round.

In a volume entitled *Letters and Papers from Prison,* Dietrich Bonhoeffer has categorically but more or less aptly and succinctly measured the character of man as a function of self-determination: "It is the characteristic excellence of the strong man that he can bring momentous issues to the fore and make a decision about them. The weak are always forced to decide between alternatives they have not chosen for themselves."

So much said, try to look inside, not to others.

Chapter 7

THE SADNESS OF PAIN

"Our aches and pains conform to opinion.
A man's as miserable as he thinks he is."

SENECA

Depression is, most probably, humanity's oldest disease. Called melancholy by Hippocrates, and described by cultures as ancient as the Assyrians', it is one of our oldest companions. As the world's oldest disease, it stands equally culpable with the world's oldest profession in keeping more people on their back than any other condition.

Depression is so protean in its presentation that it is impossible to describe it fully here. Vast texts are written on small aspects of depression. It is, however, strikingly present in persons suffering from persistent pain. It may have been present before the pain began, the pain then becoming the focus for a previously pervasive but unformed despondency. It may occur as the result of years of gnawing pain, frustration, and anger. The signs of depression include:

- A sense of hopelessness. All looks bleak. Life appears to be a long tunnel with no end in sight.
- A sense of helplessness. Depression breeds a feeling of impotence. Depressed people feel that they are powerless, that their efforts are in vain and insufficient to change their lives.
- A sense of worthlessness. Depression confers on its unwilling victims the certainty that they are without merit or virtue. They are convinced that most other people are their betters, and that no

matter what efforts they make, they will never be regarded as worthy.

■ Sleep disturbance. Either difficulty in falling or staying asleep or awakening very prematurely. This is often accompanied by disturbing dreams, a sense of dread, and a nocturnal restlessness.

■ Eating disturbance. Usually lack of appetite but at times an over-stimulation of appetite.

■ Sexual disorder. Usually the depressed person will not be able to be stimulated enough to have sex, or the act itself becomes a tedious chore rather than a pleasure.

■ Confusion. A state of mental haziness in which logical or orderly thought is difficult.

■ Mood disorder. Sadness, blueness, or tearfulness ensue. The world appears monotone and interest in most activities wanes or disappears. Interest in life may become so thin that the person wishes he were "not around." At times this leads to suicidal feelings. Usually, however, it is manifested in a heaviness or pall, an isolation and withdrawal sometimes so complete that it becomes overwhelming.

Whether depression is present before or is a consequence of the pain, the cycle is set up. Pain magnifies the depression, and depression magnifies the pain. The vortex can pull the pain victim so far down that professional counseling is needed to pull him back up.

Compounding the vortex effect is the fact that many drugs used to treat pain can themselves produce depression. Valium, often used as a muscle relaxant, often produces a mood change and a slowing of thinking. Librium, used to decrease the anxiety of pain, can produce spells of uncontrollable weeping. Steroids such as cortisone, used to relieve the inflammation of chronic pain, can often produce psychosis or severe depression. Narcotics can alter mood as well as pain. Paradoxically, then, the use of so-called pain-killers can bring on a state of sadness and depression. The Greek terms for "pain-free" (*anodynia*) and "unable to feel pleasure" (*anhedonia*) even sound and appear similar.

Two short anecdotes from our practice will help to illustrate the devastating effects of depression and chronic pain.

Paul Jacoby, the father of two small children, had been passed over for promotion at the bank twice now in five months. Although he reported to work as an assistant loan officer each day, his fellow workers and supervisors noted a lack of interest in his work and a gradual, but noticeable, isolation. He no longer ate lunch with his fellow workers, and often work was left on his desk at the end of the day. His wife, too, noticed a change. Paul had been interested in life —in the children, in school projects he had helped to build, in the care of the house, and in his lifelong involvement with sports. Lately, all of these had lost importance to Paul, and he spent many of his waking hours in bed.

Lately, too, he had begun to complain very often of a nagging backache. It had begun as a small sprain while mowing the lawn one day, but had grown into a major complaint. There even came times when Paul would refuse social invitations, saying that he hurt too much. Lately, too, he had begun to take more sick time for his back, and doctor visits were becoming routine. The spiral was beginning. Slow, chronic depression had deepened and spiraled into a pain cycle that threatened to swallow Paul and his family.

Lisa Norman underwent two back operations and was left with the knifelike stab of sciatica. The sciatica had been a constant companion down the back of her right leg since the second operation. For two years she had been seeking respite from the pain. The frustrations of daily doctor visits and physical therapy without results broadened and deepened into the full-blown syndrome of depression. She lost twenty pounds and was unable to sleep; her temper grew shorter as her relationship with her family grew more distant and ill tempered. Frequently oscillating between fighting with her family and withdrawing to her bedroom, Lisa and her family were threatened with the same uncontrolled pain-depression cycle as Paul and his family.

We can say that Paul's depression came first and his pain second, and we can point to the reverse situation for Lisa. In reality it doesn't matter. Both patients, along with their families and friends, were entering the endless cycle of chronic pain.

Are You Depressed?

The following ten questions are designed to assess depression. Answer with a simple yes or no.

1. Are you constantly plagued by a feeling of guilt or shame?
2. Do minor annoyances cause you more distress than usual?

3. Have your lost your appetite?
4. Do you wake quite early in the morning and find yourself unable to fall back to sleep?
5. Do you have difficulty focusing your attention, or are you having difficulty remembering things?
6. Do you feel as if nothing were worth doing, or have difficulty motivating yourself?
7. Have you lost interest in sex?
8. If you smoke, are you smoking more than usual? If you drink, has your drinking become a problem?
9. Are you fearful something terrible is going to happen to you?
10. Have you thought about or attempted suicide?

Depression can often accompany chronic pain, but is usually only moderately severe and may respond with treatment of the pain. There are, however, depressions that are persistent and debilitating; these may specifically require professional treatment. If you have answered yes to seven or more of the above questions, you may want to ask your physician for a professional referral. Depression is a serious problem for which there are many effective and widely available treatments. A persistent depression will inhibit the benefit of even the most comprehensive pain treatment.

Perhaps the single most important thing a pain patient can do to avoid depression or minimize its debilitating effect is to seek companionship and meaningful social interaction. Patients with chronic pain are natural victims of isolation, frequently spending a good deal of time at home away from work. Isolation is the state of being alone. At first it is a physical state, but it rapidly becomes a mental state. Alone, people insidiously begin to feel ashamed, embarrassed, and confused. They begin to lose perspective on objective events in the environment and to feel helpless and misunderstood. In turmoil, they retreat to the comfort of the bed, as much to avoid pain as to soothe their mind. It becomes tempting to hide. As depression increases, it becomes easier to yield to this temptation; hence, increasing isolation.

Studies conducted at the Boston Pain Rehabilitation Center compared two groups of patients. Those in the first group were treated as single, isolated patients and had relatively little in the way of social support. The second group was composed of people who were placed into subgroups and were helped to form social networks: in other words, to be "in touch" rather than isolated. All other variables were held constant. The "in-touch" group, in which the patients were urged to communicate with others, healed faster, were better motivated, were less depressed, and expressed less painful feelings than the isolated group *by three to one*.

Sharing words. People who talk about how they feel, feel better. Articulating problems, saying what you feel out loud with other people in the room, forces a person to understand himself a whole lot better.

Group interaction is an important aspect of our pain program. We have stressed it because it works to alleviate isolation, reduce the incidence of serious depression, and actually accelerate the process of healing. Being part of a "group" is often frightening to many new patients. Understandably, people are afraid of the unknown. We hope to encourage the reluctant pain patient to consider participation in some of the group experiences, if this form of treatment is locally available. Try it. It may help.

REFLECTIONS ON THE PAIN GROUP

They met regularly at 10 A.M. on Tuesday mornings. Al Packard would stop at the doughnut shop on the way in from College Park and bring an assortment of glazed, unglazed, and chocolate doughnuts. Dolores Fields was sure to arrive fifteen minutes early to brew a fresh pot of coffee. Fred Botley unstacked the chairs in the waiting room to ensure sufficient seating. Everyone had a part to play in getting ready.

Initially, the idea of group therapy for pain patients turned everyone off. "You mean I have to listen to other people's problems? I have enough of my own." Or "How can I possibly help anyone else? I can't manage my own pain." Or the infamous "How is talking possibly going to help my stiff back?"

Nonetheless, we encouraged everyone to join the group. While we could not guarantee success, everyone who gave the group a fair chance seemed to benefit. People liked being in the group. The sharing experience, putting feelings and ideas into words, was therapeutic: it made the pain less threatening. Being disabled by chronic pain creates stimulus starvation. Generally people find themselves sitting alone at home resting, healing, basically *waiting* to get well. The routine can be treacherous. No one is able to sleep well, at least not at night. Pacing, tossing and turning, sitting up reading, or watching TV test patterns into the wee hours were common problems. When sleep finally came, usually just before dawn, everyone else at home was preparing to wake and meet a new day. Sleeping at the wrong time kept the pain sufferer off balance, out of step with everyone else at home. The sufferer was coming when everyone else was going. After sleeping fitfully until noon, breakfast would merge into lunch. Days would be spent watching TV, waiting for family members to return, or just sitting.

The goal of the group was for each member, with the help of others, to create a personal strategy for mastering the problem of persistent pain. Having a common problem unified the members: persistent pain, be it headache, backache, migraine, or arthritis, is a great equalizer. The collective task of creating a plan for pain control relieved the stress, and for many the embarrassment, of having to talk about themselves. The lowering of defenses enabled the group to develop a cohesive structure and an intensely protective environment.

Fearing the Worst, Fear Is the Worst

For weeks Alan Klein sat silently. He listened, obviously interested in what others said, but he never spoke. Alan was quite into himself.

He always came prepared—a small memo pad which fit neatly into his shirt pocket, a pen, and a large case which he rarely opened but never let out of his sight. He sat solemnly in the group of eight staring at his pad, reviewing lists of things he had written down but didn't have the courage to discuss. Alan never put his pad down; he sat, transfixed, as if glued to his seat.

Most of the others ignored Alan, feeling that when he was ready, he would contribute. But Alan bothered Ellen Bower. His self-absorption made her uneasy.

"Alan," she exclaimed, "what the hell do you have on that pad? You've sat there for a month staring at it. Tell us what you're thinking!"

Instead of being upset or defensive, Alan appeared to welcome Ellen's challenge. He had been waiting for someone to give him permission to speak. He was not of an assertive persuasion. You had to push him to get started.

Slowly he took his eyes off his pad and looked up at Ellen. She stopped, a bit taken by his serious glance. She thought that in her impulsive haste she had upset him. She glanced at other group members for signs of support. Matt Henderson broke the silence by advising Alan that it was okay, he didn't have to talk until he felt ready. There was no pressure to make him do what he didn't want to.

Alan looked relaxed. He sighed, sat back, and thanked Ellen for her encouragement. Not prone to excesses or exaggeration, he spoke slowly and distinctly in carefully constructed sentences.

"I appreciate the group's openness. I have never been a very open person; it's difficult for me to speak in public. When I was a kid, I kept things to myself a lot. I always felt people weren't much interested in what I thought or felt or dreamed. This group made me feel differently. I feel it's safe to talk here. I had this dream I would like to share. In it, I am dead. My pain never ended. But I died. I became very tired in the dream, I went to sleep in a large bed. My arms and legs were weak. The pillows were closing around my face. It was like being suffocated by the pain.

"I have always been terrified by the idea of pain. From the first time I started having neck problems, I assumed the worst. I thought I had cancer. I would anticipate the day the doctor would finally diagnose me."

This dream was heavy. The group was silent. People were a bit uneasy. Their silence was not so much a sign that they wanted Alan to continue as fear of stopping him.

"I fervently believed there was something dreadfully wrong with my body. No matter what the specialists said, it didn't relieve my doubt. They had put me through every imaginable test."

Ellen interrupted, "Alan, didn't you have a myelogram? Didn't that help relieve your doubt that there was no serious injury?"

"I didn't believe they ever did a myelogram," he replied.

"But you told us you had one done."

"I did, but I never really believed they did it. They showed me the films but it didn't change the way I felt. No matter what they told me, it didn't matter: you see, I believed I had something terrible wrong, so whatever they told me didn't matter."

Alan's comments obviously troubled the group. Discussions of his denial were threatening to the members. Having a mental case in the group wasn't part of the deal and tonight Alan was sounding very strange.

Unable to accept Alan's blanket denial, Matt Henderson persisted. "What do you mean, the doctor didn't do the test? You were awake. You felt them stick the needles in your back, didn't you?"

"I know all that, but it didn't matter," Alan replied. "You see, I already had my mind made up."

Alan finally appeared ready to reveal his fears. "I don't understand my pain. How can someone hurt the way I hurt, day in and day out, without having a serious illness? Every time I went to a doctor and they failed to find something I was certain they were hiding the worst from me. I believed something awful was wrong and when you feel a certain way, it's hard to be convinced otherwise. Even though I know intellectually that Dr. Blakeman did the myelogram, I don't *believe* he really did it. I know that sounds crazy, but I still don't believe it."

Alan was not crazy. He was under enormous stress, and the constant burden of pain had forced him to create a series of beliefs to help him understand his condition.

"I have this recurring dream. It scares the hell out of me. In the dream I die. My death comes as a great surprise to everyone. When they review the autopsy, they discover I have a terrible disease. Everyone is astonished. The doctors are embarrassed. Finally they believe me, they realize the pain wasn't in my head."

Suddenly, Alan wept uncontrollably. "The damn pain wasn't in my head. It was real . . . it was real . . . it was real. . . ."

Alan couldn't believe he had pain without illness so he had to *believe* he was ill, and the stress of creating illness was making him sick, *emotionally* ill. The stress made his neck pain worse. He was constantly in spasm.

For many people obsessed with the fear of cancer or serious disease, it is far more creditable, even honorable, to have serious illness than live with the uncertainty and fear of constant pain. Being physically ill and fearing the worst, even being assured of the worst, is salvation. Endless reassurances only enhance the anxiety—because the pain persists. Negative finding are disregarded. Only the positive indicators of disease can quench the desire for the "real evidence" that will relieve the stress of uncertainty.

The Closeness of Pain

Ellen Pearl was so severely disabled by abdominal cramping that her internist was convinced she had regional enteritis (a severe, ulcerative disease of the small bowel that can produce extreme pain and cramping). After an extensive medical work-up failed to demonstrate active bowel disease, alternative explanations of her pain were sought. It was found that whenever Ellen was under increased stress, when the conditions of her life changed sufficiently to create anxiety, time pressures, or feelings of urgency, Ellen's bowels became hyperactive. She had explosive bouts of diarrhea and gas and was bedridden with cramping and severe pain. She would sometimes require two or three days to recuperate. The pain bouts all but ruined her social life. She was extremely self-conscious. The cramps made her feel bloated, fat, and ugly. She would not date anyone she did not know and only reluctantly went out with her friends and acquaintances, embarrassed to have them see her in her debilitated state.

She thoroughly enjoyed her work as a buyer for the juniors department of a large department store. However, any pressure (such as being late, having to meet deadlines, confronting a grouchy merchandiser) created spasms in her stomach and intensified her pain. Fortunately, her supervisor, an understanding and compassionate man, would step in and bail her out. He would spend time doing her work. Ellen felt guilty allowing him to extend himself, often to the point where he was stressed and harassed himself. She had little choice, however: without his efforts, she would surely have lost her job. Her guilt was enormous and it made her very uncomfortable. She couldn't stand being a bother to people.

Ellen joined the pain group after her internist felt that psychological factors were exacerbating her pain. Ellen spoke freely in the group. Frequently, she manipulated the sessions, but she was a friendly and outgoing woman and the group seemed to respond favorably to her. She spoke openly of psychological issues, much more so than other members. She focused on her guilt, which had its origin in her childhood. She stated that she had been a colicky and sick child who spent a good deal of time recuperating in bed. Ellen's mother was a very warm and nurturing woman who would nurse Ellen from one crisis to another. She spoke of being sick and of how guilty it made her that her mother had to spend so much of her time and attention nursing her.

Ironically, Ellen liked being a patient. It was a warm sharing between her and her mother, even though she had to be sick to enjoy it. It was a classic double bind. She was caught between wanting to be strong and healthy and to live a normal life like all the other kids, and playing the role of the sick, helpless child, nurtured by a loving and affectionate mother.

Bright, articulate, and insightful, Ellen rightly attributed the origins of her present dilemma to the mixed messages received from early childhood experiences of illness. Underneath the veneer of openness, however, she was a shy, unassuming, and painfully sensitive woman. Revealing her past as an open and dispassionate statement of personal fact was a defense against exposing her present and real self. The modern Ellen was kept hidden away.

She wanted to date, meet a nice fellow, perhaps get married someday. Although she was now struggling with a career, in the long run she saw herself a mother. Her pain left her socially frozen. She was terrified of going out with strangers for fear that a bout of diarrhea would ruin a quiet evening and embarrass her. Restaurants were off limits: eating excited her bowel too much. Dating was a dangerous and complex process, but dating, working, and socializing were only the surface of her problems. The major bind was Ellen's mother, who had cancer of the colon and was quickly losing her battle. Since the time of her illness in early childhood, Ellen's relationship with her mother had been deteriorating. Her mother's recent illness made their relationship even more difficult. Deep inside, Ellen felt responsible for her mother, in part because her mother had always taken such wonderful care of her.

"Once I got over my illness and Mother didn't spend all her time caring for me, she couldn't relate to me as a child. After having spent so much time caring for me as a patient, I think she grew impatient with me, wanting me to grow up in a hurry, to become an adult and take some of the burden from her."

Ellen had never been able to express negative or hostile feelings to her mother. Quiet, reserved, and soft-spoken as an adolescent, she appeared to be the perfect child.

"I just kept everything inside. I knew my mother loved me; she just didn't like me disagreeing with her. She had a real sense of right and wrong, of what was appropriate and inappropriate, of what adults did and what children did. I never got much of a chance to rebel, to find myself; I always had to conform to what she wanted. I felt a sense of obligation to her, like somehow it was my responsibility to always please her. If she was not happy, it was my fault." She paused. The group was always very supportive of Ellen, always encouraging her to speak about her feelings. She could do what very few of the other members could, which was to speak frankly and openly from the heart and soul.

Once she was able to share her problems and found that she had support, Ellen got better quickly. She became more assertive. She began to speak out at work and set limits with her coworkers. People came up to her and told her that she was much more professional and easier to work with. She was proud of what she was doing on the job, and it seemed that the more pride she took in her work, the more effectively she thought she was functioning, the less preoccupied and disabled she was by her pain and cramping. She felt better able to handle situations and problems. Ellen got the very most out of the group. She forced them to discuss issues and feelings that were otherwise kept deep within the recesses of people's minds and hearts.

"You know, my mother is very sick; she is dying of cancer. I think my pain is a way of sharing her burden. That may sound strange to you, but I believe that. I feel that somehow it is my responsibility to share that illness with her. Some of the warmest memories I have is her sharing my illness with me. In a way, it was our very best of times together."

The group knew that Ellen spoke truth that some of them could feel but not articulate. She dealt with her feelings by putting them into words and, by so doing, made her pain a little bit more bearable and less disabling. Being able to share the experience with other people made the whole meaning of this event much more real for both Ellen and the group.

Chapter 8

THE CRISIS OF CONFIDENCE—GAINING CONTROL, MAKING CHOICES

Confidence, the ability to act based on a high degree of faith in oneself, erodes quickly when pain is always present. The anticipation of hurt and damage imparts a sense of caution that prevents bold action. Our world, with its pace set at high speed, demands a certain degree of freedom of action that cannot be mobilized when we are in pain. "Paralyzing pain" is no accidental phrase. In both a figurative and a literal sense, pain prevents motion to prevent further damage and saps the motivation to be innovative and to take risks—the personality trait we call confidence.

Expectation, anticipation, and control are three concepts that are integral to a sense of firm belief in oneself.

Expectation is the outcome we imagine as the consequence of our actions. When we expect a favorable outcome, we take risks and, possibly, achieve. When we expect a poor outcome, we hold back. We do not achieve, but we hold our position. The person with long-term pain is always holding his position, rarely expecting that he will be successful and almost always playing a waiting game.

Anticipation is the body's way of trying to see the next moment and to prepare for it. It brings with it a tense, anxious scan of events and unconscious readjustments. Concentration is brought to bear on a problem so that all one's resources can be focused on it, as if through a magnifying glass. The person with chronic pain has fewer resources available to him and often finds it difficult to focus because of the distracting gnawing of pain.

Control is the catchword we use to describe being in charge and making choices. When we expect failure and anticipate loss of self-esteem, we seldom feel in control. We become passive and feel powerless to direct the course of our lives. We lose control of our destiny. Individuals with well-developed resources have learned to employ a broad and adaptive repertoire of coping strategies that help them retain their mastery over their environment. When pain intrudes, the process is interrupted and that quality we call confidence —"mastery over our environment"—can dissipate. The loss of control is perceived and anxiety is added to the brew, beginning a downward spiral. If we look at each of these three components, however, a pattern emerges that can turn the spiral and restore shattered confidence.

Expectation, as common to us all as breathing, can often influence the outcome of events in our lives. Expectation can fuel our hopes and, at times, our fears. The quality of our expectations determines the quality of our actions. When we expect a blow, we stiffen to ward it off. When we expect a kiss, we pucker. When we don't get it, we pout. Often, the person who expects to feel pain feels more pain than the person who has no such expectations.

Two separate experiments were done to measure the effects of expectation on surgery and the postsurgical course. One was done by Dr. Irving Janus, a psychologist at Yale, and one by us at the Hospital for Special Surgery in New York. Both experiments were designed to answer the question, "Does an expectation of disability prolong the course of recuperation after an operation, and, if so, can this be changed?" In both experiments, patients were randomly divided into two groups. In the first, they were simply observed before surgery and after surgery. Three things were measured:

1. The time it took for the wound to heal;
2. The time it took for the person to get back to work; and
3. The amount of postoperative pain experienced by the patient.

In the second group, the same three parameters were measured, but prior to surgery each patient had a one-hour talk with the examiner about the surgery, its complications, and what to expect after the operation. In both experiments, in those patients who were "prepared" and in whom expectations were taken out of the realm of guesswork, the wound healed in an average of seven days, as compared to ten days for the control groups. The time elapsed before returning to work was seven to ten days shorter than in the other groups, and the amount of postoperative pain was five points lower on a scale of one to ten. Why? Expectation is much like anticipation and uncertainty: it breeds anxiety. Anxiety, when appropriate, helps the body; when prolonged, it retards healing, delays functioning, and promotes pain.

Anticipation is a defense against the next moment, an attempt by the body to be prepared for an expected blow. Sometimes this is effective. Other times, there would be far less of a "next blow" if there were less anticipation. Think of the deer standing absolutely still in anticipation of the hunter's bullet or of the attack of a lion.

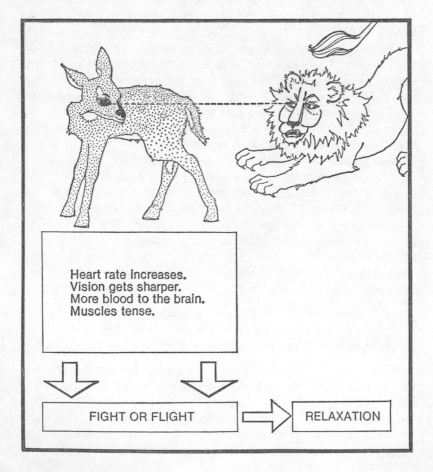

Heart rate increases.
Vision gets sharper.
More blood to the brain.
Muscles tense.

FIGHT OR FLIGHT   RELAXATION

Stress reaction and recovery.

The deer responds to an external threat by pumping adrenaline, which makes his heart throb faster, tenses his muscles, diverts blood to his brain, concentrates his vision, and makes him ready to flee or to fight. When the external danger is over, so is the reaction, and the deer can "relax." Humans, too, have the capacity for either fight or flight but, unlike animals, we have a much greater capacity for memory and the ability to respond to internal threats. Unlike the hunter's bullet or the leap of a lion, the memories associated with previously experienced threats can last a long time, leaving little opportunity for the body and the mind to relax. Thus, we are perpetually on guard for the next threat, though it never comes.

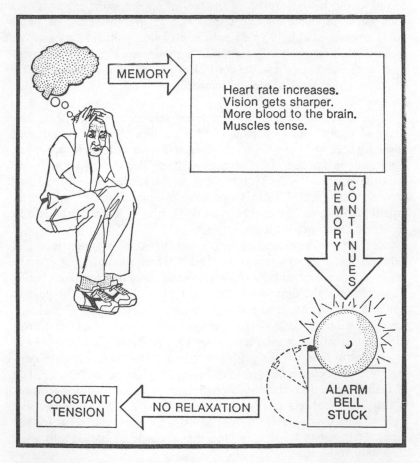

MEMORY

Heart rate increases.
Vision gets sharper.
More blood to the brain.
Muscles tense.

MEMORY CONTINUES

ALARM BELL STUCK

CONSTANT TENSION

NO RELAXATION

Chronic stress: the constant alarm.

Chronic pain patients suffer from this "alarm bell that's stuck." They are always ready for the next threat, the next muscle twist, the next ache. What is usually not understood, though, is that anticipation, with its accompanying muscle strain (as in our deer), will increase pain.

Most people are willing to accept pain they inflict upon themselves. That is, they will work in their garden for a day and accept two days of pain because they did what they liked and were able to say, "I am going to control this. I will make a choice. I will trade off working in the garden for two days of pain," or "I will sail for three hours and accept a day's pain for that." But when the pain is perceived as out of their realm of control of choice, pain angers them. This anger produces muscle spasm, which greatly increases pain. Some sources of this inflicted pain are obvious, others less so. We often think of work as inflicted upon us; there are deadlines we must meet over which we have no control. Many of us also feel that the decisions about work are in the hands of some other person and thus we are "slaves to our destiny."

If we look carefully at this reasoning, we must realize that very often we choose our own method of work. We choose our jobs, we choose where we want to work. Even if we do not, there are often deadlines we impose upon ourselves; these deadlines are as much in our control as the decision to work in the garden or sail the boat. One must ask oneself, "Am I imposing an unreasonable deadline on myself? Do I have free choice in working at my job? Did I have free choice in choosing my type of work?"

Generally, we have made a choice to work at a particular job. The pain we feel may not come at a time when we have consciously made a decision to make a trade-off (such as sailing for pain), still, we have made the decision to do that type of work, and the pain is not inflicted but comes as a necessary part of that work. We can extend this kind of deductive reasoning to other areas of our lives, such as recreation, family, and other responsibilities where we have more control than we are willing to admit. If we have ultimate control over our destiny, pain is never really inflicted on us. The essence of feeling less anger and more confidence is to feel more in control —that is, to feel less passive and more decisive. The more decisive we feel, the less anger we feel at having our lives controlled for us; the less puppetlike we feel, the less that anger is translated into muscle spasm and further pain.

Ask yourself the following questions:

1. Do I find myself angry at work when asked to finish a task by a certain time?

2. Do deadlines worry me, and do I often feel a tightness in my back and neck or my stomach as the deadline approaches?

3. Do I feel that I have no control over my work?

4. Do I feel that I have little control over my family?

5. When asked to do a difficult job either at school, at work, or at home, do I automatically feel I cannot do it well, and do I become resentful?

6. Is recreation difficult to plan? Do I have difficulty relaxing?

7. Do I feel that life controls me and not the other way around?

8. When I plan an activity, do I feel my pain is an equal trade-off for enjoyment; when others plan an activity, do I shrink back and become resentful because I know I will not enjoy it?

If most of the answers are yes, remember that these issues could produce enormous amounts of tension, muscle spasm, and pain. What is more, in many instances these outlooks could be turned around. You can have the control to make a trade-off, just as with two hours of sailing for three hours of pain. You can change the deadlines, control the situations to your advantage. In this way you can have control, do a better job, and experience less pain.

An example will illustrate this point. Paul Burton worked for a large computer firm. He enjoyed sailing, gardening, and tennis. He also had a chronically weak back, which at times gave him some trouble. He had learned, however, over the years, to trade off a day's back trouble if he really felt he wanted to plant his geraniums or to play a game of mixed doubles. There are trade-offs in life and Paul had made peace with this fact.

Three months before he came to us, Paul had been transferred to a new position with the company. He was given a task that had caused two previous supervisors to leave the company and had generated immeasurable dissension in his branch. A deadline of six months from the date of his transfer was set by the home office for completion of the project. Twelve-hour days and seven-day weeks produced strain that was more insidious and pervasive than two hours of tennis. Paul experienced increasingly intense and disabling pain as he began to get involved with the job. Working against impossible odds, he fell further behind as his back pain caused him to miss time from work. He felt he would become a failure. Becoming depressed, he felt that he would explode. He considered quitting or even removing himself by a disability retirement.

Seeking help, Paul recognized several things. First, the nature of the job was difficult—too difficult for one manager. Another manager and a new unit of clerical help had to be brought in. Second, Paul became aware that the home office vice-president had no knowledge of the complexity of the job and had just assumed that every manager was incompetent. Third, he realized that the consumer for whom the project was intended did not really need the product until the next summer. The push for completion came from the operating manager, again at the home office, and was set to further the career of the manager, not to satisfy the customer.

Paul took matters into his own hands. He exercised *control*. First, he confronted the manager and the vice-president with these facts. A crew supervisor and a clerical unit were added. Second, he confronted the vice-president with the complexity of the job and, after visiting the consumer, informed him that the deadline was unreasonable and unnecessary. After a meeting, a consensus was achieved, whereby the deadline was shifted back six months. This was an easily reachable goal. Now, with the proper help, support from above, and a reasonable deadline, Paul not only worked normal days but went to work with a sense of accomplishment and challenge. His back pain subsided. He had exercised control where he had thought none existed. If he chose to work longer hours, it was mostly his choice. He could trade off work for some increased pain *on his terms*.

Not every situation can be handled as well or as easily as Paul's. Every situation, however, in which we find outselves locked and seemingly without control can be analyzed in the fashion of Paul Burton. Many times, the increased measure of control we can assume will save days of lying in bed. If we list the mechanisms Paul used, we find that he:

- Identified the nature of his task. Any task, be it at work, at home, or socially, can be broken down into elements such as goals, resources, time allotted, supports, etc.
- Recognized that the problem in completing the task was not his alone. The two previous managers had failed partly because they took on the task themselves without acknowledging that the job was impossible for one person to do. Their confidence eroded as they fell further behind because they persisted in the belief that it was completely their responsibility.
- Understood that his predisposition to back pain was a potential liability if he overloaded himself and thus made sure he rested enough.
- Confronted those around him with whom he had contact—the

people in his "system"—and, before beginning the project, mapped out a direction as clearly as possible.

■ Created a program where uncertainty and a tendency toward self-blame were at a minimum.

Paul Burton, by exercising as much personal control as possible, reduced the uncertainty, fear of failure, and anticipation of turmoil to a minimum. His confidence returned quickly, and he was successful at his task. Had he not taken control, his back pain most assuredly would have. Had that happened, his confidence would have eroded totally and he would have failed.

The lessons learned from Paul Burton's success at work could be applied as well to social, recreational, and family interactions. Long-term pain can be a factor in grinding down endurance, eroding confidence, and producing expectations of failure. The institution of Paul Burton's principles can reverse that trend.

Chapter 9

HOW YOUR PERSONALITY MAY BE
CHANGING AND WHAT TO DO ABOUT IT

"How do you tell your family you would really like to die? . . .
Whenever we sit down together I feel I am going to come apart and
cry. . . ." *An anonymous pain patient*

Strange things happen to people under the stress of chronic pain.
During the course of treatment, a good number of our patients at
one time or another observe significant changes in their personalities. They feel differently about themselves and notice that their
relationships with other people have often taken a turn for the
worse. Pain and the problem of trying to control it has changed their
personalities.

Many, like the patient quoted above, experience isolation and intense despair but keep their feelings buried. They fear that uttering
those thoughts would hurt the ones they love most dearly. Each
passing day it becomes increasingly difficult to break the silence and
communicate. The result is tragic: people unwittingly become en-
trapped in their own internal worlds of destructive fantasy. The clarity of one's perception, unless regularly honed on the stone of personal contact and communication, is blunted.

As a general rule, people with pain do not fall apart or fragment.
Most bear the burden with stoic resolve and determination. Yet invariably, over time, characteristic changes mar the potential range of
personality. We have identified and will discuss certain patterns that
characterize the personality changes commonly seen in chronic pain
states. First, however, let us examine the concept of personality and
the attributes of sound mental health.

ON MENTAL HEALTH

Personality is unique and individual. What is right for one person is awkward and difficult for someone else. There is no one right way to be. Each person, by virtue of a particular genetic makeup, developmental experiences, mental attitude, intelligence, and aptitude, is marvelously well differentiated. Perhaps more than anything else in life, it is personality that distinguishes our originality, creativity, and diversity.

Becoming a person, developing maturity, wisdom, and, most importantly, self-acceptance, does not require changing your personality. Maturation entails becoming more fully aware of the vast potential for thought and feeling that exists internally and then allowing yourself to exercise that potential and enjoy life.

The following qualities are often considered the foundations of sound mental health:

FLEXIBILITY

The ability to shift gears fluently and effortlessly, to allow yourself to go from being happy and outgoing to serious and introspective as the situation requires. Being flexible is not the same as being easygoing, a so-called light touch or easy mark. Quite the contrary. The truly flexible individual is not easily taken advantage of for he is able to change gears and perspectives rapidly and is hence likely to get a fuller, more realistic and well-informed perspective on a situation and, in the end, react more appropriately, compassionately, and productively to changes in his environment.

PERSISTENCE

Nothing in life comes easily. Hard work, some intelligence, and genuine effort are prerequisites for the successful completion of any significant task. Of even greater value is the ability to apply these characteristics uniformly and consistently over time. Nothing is more prone to failure than inconsistent partial efforts.

CONFIDENCE

A view that one possesses sufficient internal resources to overcome adversity and prove ample to the task at hand is a personality asset of extreme importance. *Believing that you can do what others cannot is the essence of success.* Tempering that belief with a realistic assessment of your genuine talents and assets, as well as recognizing the conditions imposed by your genuine liabilities, will help present you as an effective and productive member of society.

SELF-ESTEEM

Feeling well and proud of oneself goes hand in hand with having confidence. In fact, one cannot have real confidence without maintaining the highest regard for oneself; not bravado, grandiosity, or selfishness, but simply a genuine sense of respect for oneself. Pride in one's family, appearance, job, and moral values are all part of the self system. A solid feeling of self-esteem is at the heart of the healthy personality.

CONCERN

A real sense of concern about the human condition, predicated on the sanctity and value of life, should guide the mature personality. Recognizing that life is difficult, its rewards hard won, and its stresses formidable, makes functioning humanly and empathetically a bit easier.

DIFFERENTIATION OF INNER FANTASY FROM EXTERNAL REALITY

The healthy person is endowed with a rich and imaginative fantasy world. The dreams and daydreams that provide momentary relaxation and revitalize our senses, as well as our conscious wishes, hopes, and prayers, are elements of this "inner reality."

The ability to use these inner goals as a stimulus for real-world achievement while maintaining a separateness of inner and outer reality is vital to a healthy personality. Boundaries and divisions separating the real from the unreal, the genuine from the imagined, and the possible from the impossible are critical features of sound mental health.

INTEGRATION

Over time, the various components of the personality grow and mature. The psychological defenses become more sophisticated and versatile. A sense of humor, responsibility, concern, and the capacity for love take form and substance. Insight into the self is developed. Distortions of reality are minimal and one is able to cope with painful experiences. One element essential to mental health is the integration of all of these factors—the harmonious juxtaposition of intense, diverse, and often conflicting wishes, hopes, feelings, drives, and traits into a comprehensive whole, the welding together of diverse elements into a complete self. We commonly speak of the healthy person as one who "has it all together" and is able to keep it together under the stress and strain of daily living.

CHRONIC PAIN AND PERSONALITY

Chronic pain can inadvertently destroy the potential for personality development. The constant strain of coping with pain distracts energy from other mental tasks. Pain creates a reallocation of mental energy resources, depriving the healthy personality of the energy necessary to accomplish normal tasks of development. Consequently, the events of daily living that most of us take for granted become burdensome. Pain keeps one home from work, out of sports competition, uninvolved with other family members, and uninterested in social and civic functions. The person with pain has difficulty tending to the tasks of development—the famous "passages" we all go through in growing up. Energy is spent unproductively. Not only is the course of normal development altered, so is one's perspective on life.

A person with chronic pain must work harder to achieve the same goals as someone without pain. Pain strains the motivational engine. Instead of expanding and broadening the depth and scope of our personality, the chronic pain patient invariably experiences constriction and rigidity of the personality, analogous to the patient whose leg is fractured and casted: the inevitable restriction of movement creates muscle stiffness, joint restriction, and generalized body rigidity. The chronic pain personality becomes unusually one-dimensional.

This monochromatic personality lacks sufficient flexibility and resources to handle the full range of human stresses encountered in everyday life. The personality changes one observes in chronic pain states are caricatures that highlight and exaggerate certain predominant features; the "whole" of the person is eclipsed by a series of fragments. Highly idiosyncratic patterns of behavior predominate.

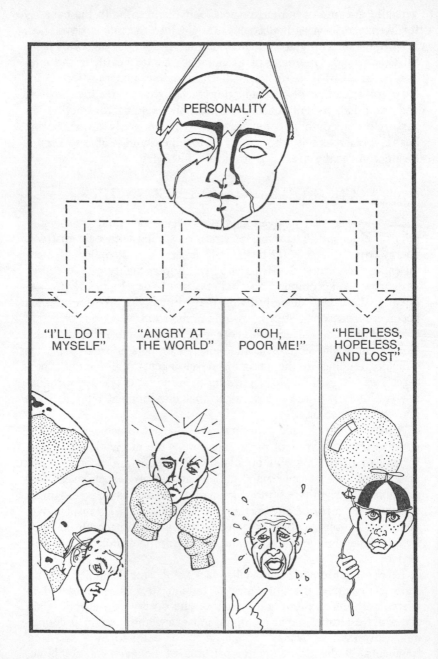

Under the stress of chronic pain, people tend to be less able to exert the full range of their personality. Consequently, the most accessible elements and the most highly practiced parts of the personality are used excessively; for example, the rigid individual becomes increasingly rigid while the angry, explosive person may show less and less capacity to control his anger.

Patterns of Departure

For the purpose of illustration, we have arbitrarily delineated four major personality subgroups. While not everyone whose personality is affected by chronic pain will fall into one of these four groups, the categories represent a psychological model for organizing the response to pain. Our design is not intended to be all-inclusive or scientifically exact, but merely to illustrate certain common pathways of personality disorganization. The figure above represents, graphically, the disorganizing effect of pain on the personality and the possible departures from the norm.

SELF-EXAMINATION

For each personality type we have designed a small quiz. For each quiz, please answer the ten questions and then score the test by awarding five (5) points for an answer you *strongly agree* with, four (4) points for an answer you simply *agree* with, three (3) for *undecided,* two (2) for *disagree,* and one (1) for *strongly disagree.*

QUIZ NO. 1

Am I the Man or Woman Who Will Do It by Myself?

SA A U D SD

1. I hate being dependent on the people I live with. — — — — —
2. I usually hold back, actively restrain myself from letting anyone know anything about my pain. — — — — —

SA A U D SD

3. I feel embarrassed and ashamed when
   people notice my poor health.   __ __ __ __ __

4. I put my family through so much I do not
   understand how they can still love me.   __ __ __ __ __

5. I do not consider myself to be sick or
   disabled even though I am in almost
   constant pain.   __ __ __ __ __

6. Anything that can be done for me has
   already been tried.   __ __ __ __ __

7. If others could feel my pain they would
   understand me a lot better.   __ __ __ __ __

8. I would prefer to work even with great
   pain rather than allow someone else to
   do my job.   __ __ __ __ __

9. I cannot accept help without feeling
   humiliated.   __ __ __ __ __

10. Sometimes I get so caught up with myself
    that I lose touch with my family.   __ __ __ __ __

QUIZ NO. 2

Am I Angry with the World?

SA A U D SD

1. Medical and surgical failures are
   responsible for my pain.   __ __ __ __ __

2. Often I do not know what to do about
   my pain and my doctors give me
   confusing information.   __ __ __ __ __

3. As a child it was important to protect
   myself from all my enemies.   __ __ __ __ __

4. The right doctor could cure my pain.   __ __ __ __ __

5. Sometimes I wonder how people can
   possibly stand me.   __ __ __ __ __

6. I don't believe people take my pain
   seriously enough.   __ __ __ __ __

SA A U D SD

7. A doctor should do every possible test
   to be absolutely certain that he is not
   missing something.   — — — — —
8. I do not deserve to be in pain.   — — — — —
9. I have problems controlling my temper;
   my fuse seems to be getting shorter as
   I get older.   — — — — —
10. I am a very difficult person to get along
    with since I have been in pain.   — — — — —

QUIZ NO. 3

Am I The "Oh, Poor Me!" Self-Pitier?

SA A U D SD

1. I have lost the best years of my life due
   to pain.   — — — — —
2. Pain, while uncomfortable, has become
   a familiar companion.   — — — — —
3. The last time I can remember being truly
   happy was before I became ill.   — — — — —
4. Pain is my cross to bear.   — — — — —
5. Friends tell me I spend too much time
   talking about my problems.   — — — — —
6. Since all my problems are related to my
   pain, I will be a happy person when my
   pain is relieved.   — — — — —
7. Worrying about myself keeps me from
   doing other things.   — — — — —
8. I appreciate people being sympathetic
   as it means they really care for me.   — — — — —
9. I feel good when someone recognizes my
   capacity to stand pain.   — — — — —
10. I don't believe I will ever be free of pain.   — — — — —

QUIZ NO. 4

Am I the "Helpless, Hopeless, Lost Person"?

	SA	A	U	D	SD
1. It is very difficult to have friends if you are sick.	—	—	—	—	—
2. In pain one cannot come close to anyone else.	—	—	—	—	—
3. I always feel guilty for causing problems for other people.	—	—	—	—	—
4. At times I feel utterly helpless to do anything about my pain.	—	—	—	—	—
5. It is useless to do anything more to try to improve my condition.	—	—	—	—	—
6. I frequently feel sorry for myself.	—	—	—	—	—
7. I would be afraid to try any new treatment as it might make me worse.	—	—	—	—	—
8. Since I have become ill, my family smothers me.	—	—	—	—	—
9. I often feel no one cares about me.	—	—	—	—	—
10. Pain severely limits me from doing pleasurable things.	—	—	—	—	—

SUMMARY

Tabulate your results. Remember, there are no correct and hence no incorrect answers. We are simply trying to formulate a basis for analyzing trends. If you have a score greater than forty (40) points in any particular category, you might pay careful attention to some of the following analyses.

In our practice we routinely use the Minnesota Multiphasic Personality Inventory (MMPI) for personality assessment. The test is perhaps the most widely available measure of the various normal and abnormal elements of the personality, and an important clinical tool for psychiatrists and psychologists.

From our records, we have selected four patients whose MMPI records illustrate some of the points that we have tried to make in this simplified test. We have excerpted portions of the MMPI computer profile which we feel illustrate the patterns of personality deterioration most commonly seen in the chronic pain states.

FROM THE RECORDS

PERSONALITY TYPE: "I'LL DO IT MY WAY"

"The unwillingness of this patient to admit to the relatively minor faults which most people have suggests that he is a person with a strong need to be seen by others and perhaps by himself as an unusually virtuous person. Such people tend to be naïvely defensive and uncompromising individuals who stress moral issues and emphasize their own integrity. They tend to be frustrated, insecure individuals who have little insight and are unaware of their own stimulus value.

"This patient may show a variety of physical complaints. Among these are pain which usually appears in the head, back, or neck, or symptoms involving food such as discomfort after eating and sometimes anorexia or hysterical vomiting. Although he is not likely to be incapacitated by his symptoms, they are likely to increase with emotional stress. He may have a long history of insecurity and immaturity. Despite his discomfort he does not seem greatly concerned about his emotional state and he may object to psychiatric study or treatment because of his conviction that his difficulty is entirely physical."

PERSONALITY TYPE: "ANGRY AT THE WORLD"

"This presentation of herself is deviant, and may represent a hostile, rebellious attitude toward the evaluation. Similar patterns are sometimes seen in patients who are unable to understand the items or correctly follow the instructions. If this can be ruled out, this pattern may reflect hostility, poor self-control, and a potential for aggressive acting out in a seriously disturbed person. Test subjects who are in difficulty with the law or otherwise feel coerced to control by others are particularly likely to present this picture. This test result should be supplemented by further evaluation to establish the patient's current mental status.

"This patient is a withdrawn, inhibited individual who spends a good deal of time in personal fantasies and daydreams. Her thinking tends to be unusual and unconventional. The possibility of a serious psychiatric disturbance should be carefully explored. Characteristic symptoms that might be anticipated in this patient are depression, irritability, and extreme suspiciousness. Physical complaints and medical fads may have served to stabilize the patient's precarious emotional adjustment. . . . In times of prolonged emotional stress she may develop symptoms such as headache, gastrointestinal disorders. She appears to be a person who represses and denies emotional distress. While she may respond readily to advice and reassurance, she may be unwilling to accept the psychological interpretation of her difficulties.

"She is concerned to an unusual degree with bodily functions and health. She may overreact to illness and complain unreasonably about relatively minor ailments."

PERSONALITY TYPE: "OH ME, OH MY"

"This patient apparently has an intense need to appear in good light. In an effort to prove his social conformity, he denies the minimal kinds of shortcomings which most people have and readily admit to. This suggests that he is a relatively naïve person who, because of an insecurity, lacks insight into his own behavior and denies unfavorable traits both to himself and to others. Such patients tend to be rigid, repressive individuals who are stereotypical and unoriginal in their responses to problems. They are concerned primarily with their surface image and have little awareness of their own impact on others.

"This patient may exhibit a variety of physical symptoms with an absence of overt anxiety and depression. It appears that the patient is focusing his attention and concern on bodily function and showing extreme denial of emotional problems. Frequent symptoms are pain especially in the head, chest, or stomach, problems in eating, such as loss of appetite or overeating, and insomnia.

"This patient tends to complain of minor and often trivial complaints and presents himself as needful and desirous of nurturing response."

PERSONALITY TYPE: "OH HELPLESS ME"

". . . it appears that this patient is somewhat self-critical. She may be somewhat more likely than the average person to admit to symptoms and psychological problems, even when they are minimal.

"This patient shows a personality pattern which occurs frequently among persons who seek medical or psychiatric attention. Feelings of inadequacy, sexual conflict, and rigidity are accompanied by a sense of pervasive helplessness. They experience a loss of efficiency, initiative, and self-confidence. Their self-esteem is extremely low. Insomnia is likely to occur along with chronic anxiety, fatigue, and tension. This individual may have suicidal thoughts and depression as her dominant feature. The basic characteristics are resistance to change and her symptoms tend to remain stable with time. She expresses convincing arguments that there is little she can do to help herself."

SOME FINAL COMMENTS

There are many people who will be concerned about changes in their personalities. The persistence of pain may increase irritability, decrease frustration tolerance, and increase the need for immediate gratification, thus contributing to a general loss of coping strength.

Anyone who has watched as pain attacks the mental health of a loved one can fully understand the potential problem. Pain does not cripple through physical means alone. Sometimes the most punishing handicaps are the most difficult to assess.

If you are concerned about the changes in your personality or behavior, we recommend the following:

1. Sit down with your family and have a frank discussion. Try to understand how they see you or if they have noticed changes in your personality. Often it is difficult for loved ones to share these kinds of observations for fear of hurting your feelings or upsetting you.

2. See your physician and discuss your concerns. He may also have noticed changes and may have been reluctant to discuss them with you. Invite his input.

3. Perhaps rereading the section "A Healthy Personality," above, will provide some useful insights. Clearly, there are no quick cures, but being aware of the problem is a major step in the right direction.

Chapter 10

BRITTLE HOMES AND FAMILIES AND HOW TO MEND THEM

For so many of us, the family is a refuge from the world. It is a place to rest, to relax, to be revitalized, nurtured, and fed. The family can irritate, frustrate, perplex, and abuse, but for most it represents a retreat. André Maurois, in *The Art of Living,* stated rather eloquently: "Without a family, man alone in the world trembles with the cold. A friend loves you for your intelligence, a mistress for your charm, but a family's love is unreasoning; you are born into it and are of it, flesh and blood."

If you accept the nurturing quality of most families, how is it possible for that same oasis to propagate the pain that is so distressing?

The answer lies in the duality of the family. In the nurturing atmosphere of the family lies the seed of overdependence. In its closeness, the family often lacks objectivity. Without objectivity, a sense of helplessness can develop. Because the family cares, it may begin to care too much, and frustration and resentment may build. Finally, in the family's natural desire to care for, shelter, and love its members, perspective may be lost. Inertia then takes over, and the family loses sight of the fact that it exists in the greater context of the outside world. It becomes a cocoon, oblivious to the fact that the isolation it breeds can sap its members of the ability to tolerate the frustrations of the real world.

We have identified four types of families that we have seen contribute to the pain-go-round. Usually, if the family is a unit, its members are not aware that they are anything but caring. They are shocked to learn that they contribute to distress. These four types of family are:

1. Oh Dad, Poor Dad
2. Hidden Resenters
3. Helpless Helpmates
4. Good Old Troopers

1. *Oh Dad, Poor Dad.* This family feels so bad about Dad's
pain and cares so much that in an attempt to make him feel better, it
surrounds him with enough love to drown a small army. There is no
false love here. The family members see the daily suffering of their
father (or mother) and, with the sincerity of a cleric, attempt to ex-
orcise the pain with kindness and devotion. When he hurts, they are
there. No need to get up for any creature comforts, the rest of the
family will do it. No need to do anything, because the family in its
infinite love will end the hurting.

In Japan, there is a type of beef called Kobe beef. It is the most
tender and the most expensive in the world. The cows, from infancy,
are never allowed to move. They are fed on beer and given a massage twice a day; they want for nothing. In the end, they are hit in
the head and eaten. Dad is not eaten, but sooner or later he is hit
in the head with the realization that he has forgotten the skills necessary to interact in the world. He has also missed learning the skills
necessary to deal with his pain. He has been cheated by a family too
loving and caring to give him the opportunity to care for himself.

2. *Hidden Resenters.* Paul Grant had been out of work for six
months. By receiving workmen's compensation, he was able to pay
for basic necessities. His wife, of course, worked and never minded
working. She even suggested that she get a second job to help ends
meet. Paul agreed, remarking regretfully that it was too bad that he
hurt so much that he could not help out by returning to work. His
wife, a caring and loving individual, worked two jobs and continued
to drive Paul to his physicians to get checked and worked up and
exercised.

Paul's wife did everything that a loving wife would. She never told
him about the growing resentment, the nagging anger, the fatigue at
the end of each day that made her irritable with the children. Unable to tell her husband about her feelings, she began to experience
depression. Her children noted the difference and, being children
and quite aware of things, understood the reason. Her husband
never did. He was so used to dealing with his own pain that he
could not even begin to touch upon the growing stress in his wife.
His wife, brought up to hold in her frustrations, tried to deal with

them herself. She would never tell her husband, and so they would never try to work out a system where the family could be a vehicle in which to cope rather than a time bomb that one day would explode. When that happened, the fallout in terms of physical and emotional pain set Paul's progress back years, and possibly destroyed his family. No malice was ever intended. Neither was any understanding.

3. *Helpless Helpmates.* This family, in a way, is at the other end of the spectrum. In most families, there is often one member more dependent than the others and who relies on another, the counter-dependent member, to carry out decisions. When the less dependent, more dominant member of the family becomes ill with pain, the dependent member becomes worried. He then becomes anxious, frightened, and unable to make any decisions. Always having believed in the fantasy that the spouse could "make everything right," the Helpless Helpmate is now paralyzed with the fear that functioning is going to be impossible because the mate is ill. Usually, the entire bench is called in—neighbors, friends, relatives, doctors—and the spouse ends up in a circle trying desperately to help the mate get better so that he or she can again take control of making large and small decisions.

This, of course, can go on only so long before the entire system collapses of its own weight. Neighbors have other chores; friends begin to plead that they have their own families; relatives begin to move to San Diego; and the doctor promises to move his practice to Sun City, Arizona, because, at the age of forty-one, he has had it. Meanwhile, the chronic pain patient has been lost in the shuffle and has received virtually no support or help. Quite the contrary; his supports have all moved away or have promised never to speak to him again. Usually without much understanding of why this is happening or that his mate has managed to isolate him, he scratches his head and puts on another heating pad, and his pain continues.

Unlike the Oh Dad family, the Helpless Helpmate family unknowingly removes all support from the pain sufferer. Instead of being smothered, he is abandoned, and nobody understands why.

4. *Good Old Troopers.* Good old troopers are like the infantry: they do not question, they just follow orders. They do not smother like the Oh Dad, Poor Dad group, nor do they resent. They are not helpless. They are just oblivious. The troopers have a momentum like an armored battle unit. Looking neither to the right nor to the left, the family presses on without regard to external pressures or in-

ternal cracks in the foundation. Pain is a subtle, pervasive problem, and it requires attention to nuances. The trooper's family has not looked to the right or left for years. Rigid and unbending, this family is unable to adapt to the changing needs and expectations of the pain-prone person. Unquestioning, it will appear supportive for a while, following the doctor's orders, even if it means that the patient is swallowing five different kinds of pills from four doctors.

Characteristically compliant, it would appear that this family provides the necessary care. Underneath their ministrations the rigidity of the seemingly helpful people does not allow for aberration, and so the pain victim of the family is slowly, subtly, and unwittingly left behind like the wounded soldier so that the rest of the company can move on.

Each of these family types in its particular style compromises the process of healing. Most of the members of these families would be aghast to learn that they were retarding healing instead of promoting it. They are not malicious; they believe they are doing "what is best." There is no plot, no villain. The only conspiracy is one of unwitting ignorance. Without intervention, the Oh Dad, Poor Dad family will continue to smother the patient into lasting pain; the Resenters will, by silence and anger, undermine the fabric of the supportive family; the Helpless Helpmate will leave the pain sufferer wondering why he cannot find support around him; and the Good Old Trooper will march on, leaving the pain patient behind to wonder where the rest of the family went.

What can be done to intervene? Recognition, of course, is the first step. Every patient with pain and each family of a pain victim must examine the family's ways of reacting to their situation. Is resentment covered up? Does the family march on without regard to danger signals? Is the pain patient being left behind? Is the daily routine of having a father's every need cared for smothering his ability to cope? If so, the pain-go-round is pushed a little faster each time.

Following are ten hints on family interaction that are helpful to the pain patient:

1. Family interaction, especially at mealtimes, should revolve around any activity not directly involved with pain. Talking about school or making decisions regarding which fabrics look better are perfectly legitimate and avoid the pitfall of involving the patient in the continuous activity of looking at his pain.

2. The victim of chronic pain should be allowed to act for himself, from getting the catsup out of the refrigerator to changing the channel on TV. This, of course, should be done within reason. All the leaves in the yard are not to be raked by someone with a chronic pain problem, but certainly the pain patient should be allowed to perform as much as possible for himself.

3. Feelings of anger, resentment, and frustration should be spoken about openly, and at the time of their occurrence, not two weeks later.

4. Limitations based on pain should be recognized. If Dad cannot lift the wheelbarrow anymore, the family should get together to decide how various jobs should be divided up, giving Dad the part of the job not risky or injurious to his health.

5. Patterns of help from friends, relatives, and neighbors should be assessed. If it is decided that they are making decisions for the family or doing tasks that are legitimately the family's, a shift should be made.

6. An ongoing and honest reassessment of the family's progress in overcoming pain should be made on a regular basis—once a week, for instance, and by all members of the family old enough to be affected by the pain.

7. A long-range plan, based on the family's needs, desires, limitations, and options, should be drawn up, with the expectation that the family is involved in the pain every bit as much as the identified patient. Remember young children are part of the family and should be considered when making family plans. When an adult is ill, there is a temptation to demand unusual compliance from youngsters. Children always need room to do what they do best; that is, act like children.

8. Doctors and other persons involved in the treatment of the pain should be questioned carefully, keeping in mind that consistency of treatment means not only that the doctors and nurses should be consistent, but that the family should be internally so as well.

9. The family should become acquainted with the effects and side effects of all medications. When Mom is groggy at noontime, the family needs to be able to communicate to the doctor that there is an unwanted side effect. At times Mom will not be able to do so.

10. Help the pain sufferer help himself. Each member of the family should be open and receptive enough to be able to say "No, you cannot do that," as well as "I'll help you with that; I know that at this stage you cannot." Asserting yourself, especially to someone who is not feeling well, requires confidence. Practice makes perfect.

III

GETTING OFF THE
PAIN-GO-ROUND:
CREATING A PERSONAL
PAIN CONTROL PROGRAM

Chapter 11

GETTING WELL IS AN ACTIVE PROCESS

Before conceiving a treatment program for pain, we developed a treatment philosophy. Simply stated, we believe that every person must accept a certain critical measure of responsibility for the control of his pain. The better able we are to encourage, educate, and ultimately motivate people to share with their physicians the responsibility for getting well, the more complete the pain control.

Our philosophy is based on the following three factors, each of which is critical in influencing not only the eventual recovery from pain but also the potential for disability. First, the growth of technology in modern medical practice is beginning to outstrip the capacity for the humanistic application of principle. Second, the need to "treat" people, to assume an inordinate and at times excessive responsibility for their recovery, has infringed on "patient rights" and created an unrealistic public expectation for complete and immediate care. The availability and accessibility of "good health care" has created an urgency to be well that can interfere with the natural process of healing. Finally, we believe that pain is a critical symptom signaling disturbance in the body's natural system of defense against disease. Pain is a message indicative of body malfunctioning. Understanding pain's message, recognizing it as an expression of "disordered homeostasis," is critical to recovery.

PATIENTLESS MEDICINE

During the nineteen-eighties, Americans may face a new crisis in health care: patient obsolescence. The geometric escalation of electronic technology has already brought us through several decades of vocational, computer, and educational obsolescence. Things get old very fast. A recent business article noted that MBAs who graduated in 1979 found that fully 80 percent of their "technical education" was outdated and hence inapplicable in 1981, just two years after graduation. We may be locked into the involuntary process of making patients themselves unnecessary.

If communication technology grows at its current rate of unmolested escalation, by 1990 we may experience a renaissance in health care. Conceivably, health care can be done aseptically and electronically from the comfort of one's home. Imagine becoming ill, being diagnosed, and subsequently receiving treatment without having to hassle crowded waiting rooms, endless phone calls (sitting on hold), and chilly examining rooms. Can we eventually progress to the point of making the patient extraneous? Is it desirable to remove human input, fraught with inconsistency and emotional bias, from the diagnostic and therapeutic process? Will technological treatment based on "hard data"—the real stuff of computerized scans, blood and organ fluid levels, and the physiological profile of normal function, ultimately regulate the process of health care?

Sound absurd? The idea of computerized health care is not ridiculous, it is operative. Computerized health assessments have infiltrated all areas of medicine from radiology to psychiatry. Computers are extensively utilized in the training of medical students. Increasingly, numerous aspects of care, ranging from the creation of medical records to assessment of differential diagnosis, are being programmed in computers.

Modern therapy, filled with the technological wizardry and sophisticated discoveries of the past twenty-five years, has to a large measure obviated the need for extensive personal inquiry. Students of medicine are obsessed with scientific facts. The amount of information that can be obtained from X rays, laboratory data, and electronic data is mind-boggling. Seeing the patient, comforting and supporting the person, is for many physicians a secondary concern. My wife, who as a nurse witnesses the doctor-patient relationship firsthand, comments that this is a sad observation on the current state of the art. As usual, she is right. Perhaps we have access to too much information, we have become informed too rapidly, too extensively. The travail of personal history, with its hidden and uniquely personal revelation, has become an archaic symbol of old-time medicine.

Science can advance our understanding of human processes; it cannot, however, become or replace a human process. The illusion that every cause has an effect, every problem a solution, and, of course, every disease a cure, can blind us to the truth—which is that, despite all we know, we know very little.

MAKING PROGRESS

Not long ago, we came across an article describing the critical limitations and application of cardiac surgical theories. Before 1955, operating on the human heart was a major surgical procedure bordering on the experimental. Unable to stop the cardiac pulsation, the surgeon employed ingenious techniques to work around the heart, repairing only the most superficial, external, and easily accessible defects. What was required was a means of diverting the cardiac output and temporarily stopping the heart. The cardiac surgeon would flourish if only he had a "heart-lung" machine to assist him.

In 1954, the medical world community dreamed of developing such a sophisticated device. Medical reports out of a major teaching center in Boston cautioned, "The development of extracorporeal pump oxygenation (a heart-lung machine) is not going to be available in the foreseeable future." These reports were not capricious or whimsical; they reflected the consensual convictions of prominent researchers and surgeons in Boston.

Almost simultaneously, in Rochester, Minnesota, the members of a cardiac-pulmonary laboratory were committing themselves to a monumental research protocol. They had developed a heart-lung machine, a device that would allow the surgeon precious moments of undisturbed calm to open, dissect, and repair the damaged hearts of children with congenital defects. An initial series of eight patients was selected for the surgery. The Mayo team had developed and was going to use a real heart-lung machine. They succeeded, and the rest is history. Virtually every major medical center in the world today routinely does open heart surgery. The original prototype oxygenator has been grossly revamped and redesigned to be more efficient and reliable and less traumatic to the blood. Only the principle remained: a machine to replace the heart in surgery.

The world of cardiac surgery was changed in the course of several months; the field was revolutionized. Fortunately, the surgeons and the public were ready.

But can we sustain this burst of technological advances? As a nation, we nurtured and supported the growth of cardiac surgery through its inception and into its adolescence. It was novel, a gifted child judiciously placed in the forefront of priorities. The problems of growth were easily identified: if you failed to apply to technology astutely, the patient died. Survival statistics documented clinical efficacy and substantiated competence. Heart surgery assumed center stage. What people had dreamed about for decades became a reality in months, a science in years, and, ultimately, a business.

The story of cardiac surgery over the past twenty-five years details the very best of American initiative and mastery. A major break-through in technology was subtly blended with a well-researched, scientifically established, surgical expertise. The people and the machines melded in perfect unison. Everyone benefitted.

But has all medicine kept pace? Has the publicity justifiably celebrating the marvels of medicine blinded us from seeing the limitations of our real knowledge? Have we come to expect too much from the doctors and too little from ourselves?

Americans and Their Health

It has never been difficult in this country to sell people on the idea of good health care. Everyone wants the best and is willing to pay for it (or at least to allow his insurance company to pay for it). While Americans have always been superconscious of the need for top-flight diagnostic and therapeutic health measures, their zeal for top performance has rarely spread into the area of self-regulated preventive measures. Though we might spend considerable time wondering who will care for us when we are ill, we do little to protect our health. Perhaps we have been lulled into believing that the great paternalistic system of American Medicine can cure anything.

A doctor friend recently expressed concern over his perception of a growing wave of subtle yet palpable hostility among his patients. Not only do paying patients repudiate the possibility of chronic pain, but sick patients in general disavow the presence of disease. The disclaimer is often vociferous or otherwise demonstrative. People are phobic of being ill, and take the matter out directly on their physicians as if they were somehow responsible. My colleague repeats the following dialogue from rounds:

PHYSICIAN: Good morning, Mr. Barrett. How are you today?
MR. BARRETT: I still have a fever. [Harshly.]
PHYSICIAN: You do? [Momentarily taken aback, he begins to examine the patient's chart.]

MR. BARRETT: How come?

PHYSICIAN: How come what?

MR. BARRETT: How come I still have a fever? [Again, harshly.]

PHYSICIAN: [Again taken aback, pauses.] Well, you have pneumonia, Mr. Barrett. Fever is one of the symptoms of your illness.

MR. BARRETT: How do you know I still have pneumonia? Have you seen this morning's X ray?

PHYSICIAN: [Patting the patient, obviously threatened by the patient's line of inquiry.] X ray?

MR. BARRETT: Yes, my X ray. They just took another one this morning.

PHYSICIAN: No, Mr. Barrett. I haven't seen it yet. I have just begun my morning rounds.

MR. BARRETT: How come you haven't seen my X ray yet?

The dialogue is subtle. My colleague confirms that the patient's tone was angry; he was clearly shaken. As an aside, he is an excellent physician, concerned, thorough, and friendly—but not perfect.

The patient exhibits a bit of the new assertiveness popularized by the media exploitation of behavioral self-help strategies. I am afraid the self-indulgent, me-first pushiness of the nineteen-seventies has begun to affect the health consumer. We call it "patient macho."

The rights of the consumer have become part of the health care issue. Assuming that good health is part of the American heritage to which by birth and citizenship we are all entitled, one demands from physicians guidance and treatment sufficient and necessary to attain and maintain good health. We have been subtly led to believe, by such authorities as pharmaceutical manufacturers, health care administrators, and physicians concerned with the marketing of their skills and technological possessions (which are heavily mortgaged and require extensive utilization) that no one is supposed to be sick or harbor a chronic disease.

We have adapted a new entitlement—a right to the best care possible. As long as the marketers sell the best, why not demand it? A logical extension of this premise, one which has generated more referrals and repetitious and unnecessary medical tests, is the assumption that persistent pain is unwarranted and that further exploration, preferably under a guide of greater competence and expertise, will extricate the source of one's complaint. As we have shown, however, the search for the Holy Grail of a pain-free life is a tedious and debilitating journey.

Even the burden of cost does not curb our appetite for thorough investigation and exhaustive research. In the health profession, we espouse the conviction that if someone is sick he deserves the best. The decision to spend fifteen thousand dollars to explore the possibility of a brain tumor in someone with no clinical findings (the actual average cost is taken from a clinical study) is easily made, with the justification that cost is inconsequential in the quest for treatable illness. Our allocation of resources is directed at diagnosing diseases and not at creating programs of prevention. We are much more apt to respond to issues of our ill health than to encourage efforts at prevention.

We recently cautioned a patient on the ills of smoking and on the necessity of making every effort to stop while he was still young and in good health. The patient replied, "Oh, I know smoking is no good for you, Doc, but I take good care of myself." Puzzled, I questioned, "How do you care for yourself when you continue to smoke, despite overwhelming evidence on the dangers of smoking?" The patient replied, "Easy. I'm smart. I get a chest X ray every six months. The minute anything abnormal shows up, I take care of it early, before the problem gets out of hand."

For many, having the problem is already having things "out of hand." Certainly, for the smoker, noticing a small shadow on a chest film can mean a terminal cancer. Our patient was naïve, as are many Americans; he felt that if he became ill the science of medicine would surely offer him a cure. Medical science may offer relief from suffering and alleviate many diseases, but it is not omnipotent. Much more can be gained from understanding how to preserve your health than from knowing how to treat it when it is impaired.

On Waiting Around for Someone to Have a Good Idea

There is a Yiddish proverb that says, "It's good to hope; it's waiting that spoils it." One of the alternatives to doing for yourself is waiting for someone to do for you.

The following dialogue between Dr. Schulman and Al Einstein, a pain patient, illustrates how compliant and hopeful many people are when they delegate the responsibility of getting well to someone else —preferably a physician.

Dr. Schulman had a patient, Al, who had been suffering with cervical myofascial pain for many years. Everything that could be done for him was tried; still his pain persisted. He had seen numerous specialists, had undergone every conceivable diagnostic test, and had undergone a broad range of treatment—without much success. He still had his pain.

Over the three years since his injury and the onset of his pain, he had gained fifty pounds (mostly in a large belly overhanging his belt); he had given up any semblance of regular physical exercise, and had generally deteriorated physically. We had been after him for years to lose the weight, establish a regular fitness program, and begin vocational rehabilitation. Al, like many chronic pain sufferers, persisted in his efforts to find the source of his pain.

Rather inadvertently, while in the hospital for a gallbladder flare-up, he mentioned to the attending surgeon that he had pain in his neck (the same pain that had kept him out of work for three years and had led him to twenty other specialists). The surgeon, who was not familiar with Al's pain history, requested a new orthopedic surgeon to consult with Al while he was still in the hospital for treatment of his gallbladder condition.

Al made some efforts to conceal his pain history from the surgeon, as he felt the new doctor's evaluation would be biased by his long history of treatment failures. He relished the idea of an impartial opinion.

After a cursory examination and some cervical X rays that were unremarkable, the orthopedic surgeon recommended a two-week course of cervical traction. Al thought that this was a wonderful idea; after all, it was a new idea, something not previously tried. He was ecstatic; at least this doctor had something positive to offer. As he told the story, Al's eyes gleamed. "Don't you think that's a great idea, Doctor?"

"Yes. In fact, it's terrific."

A bit taken aback that Dr. Schulman, the eternal skeptic, would agree with him so readily, he queried further, "You do?"

Not quite certain he had heard correctly, Dr. Schulman responded, "Yes. I believe that being in traction is a wonderful idea —if you have an acute problem that would respond to two weeks of bed rest and traction. But I have my doubts that after three years of chronic pain you would get very much out of it."

"You mean you don't think it is a good idea?"

"Traction may be a great idea, but not for you," he remarked.

"Then why would the doctor suggest it?"

"Probably you didn't tell him the whole story, including all the treatments that you have gone through. Good ideas are easy. One that may work for you is to lose some weight. Walking around with that gut is a bit like being in 'antitraction.' Remember, your sore back has to support all that weight."

Al's wishing for a "good idea" is not unusual. There are as many as 40 million Americans with some type of chronic pain who share Al's desire for a "cure." Unfortunately, there are few, if any, cures immediately forthcoming. We hope most of those 40 million Americans are not sitting around enduring the agony of chronic pain and waiting for miracles to occur. It is nice to believe in something, to have faith and hope, but it's hell waiting around for miracles.

No one is doomed to suffer endlessly. Something positive can be accomplished with motivation, determination, and a personal strategy for pain control. Al's error was that he tried to govern events to control others, rather than apply himself to the process of getting well. It is impossible to control others when one is not fully in control of himself.

Medical science can show us what is possible; we must choose what is best. If you understand what ails you, if you recognize that some pain and discomfort are inevitable, and if you can appreciate the benefits and limitations of science, the likelihood of recovery will be greatly increased.

Whom Do You Trust?

It is becoming increasingly difficult to function intelligently in the role of patient. The sheer size of our health system is overpowering. Whole cities exist as "medical centers," linked together by a labyrinthine network of tunnels connecting hospital to research center to more hospital, to outpatient clinical centers and back again. They are staffed by an enlarging army of medical specialists and paraprofessionals, who (with the aid of computer technology) program people into, through, and eventually out of the clinical compound.

As a nation, we focus political attention on the inequities of social and job discrimination on the basis of race, sex, and nationality, but we appear indifferent to the discriminatory fact that high-powered medical care services depersonalize the delivery of health care. The resilience and uniqueness of each individual is often overlooked in the stampede to offer uniformly first-rate, quality care.

Far too frequently, we minimize the difficulty involved in being a good patient. We assume that since getting sick was not a matter of choice, getting well is also a passive process. Actually, nothing could be further from the truth. Being a good patient and actually contributing to the therapeutic process of getting well is a difficult task. The temptation to sit back and allow someone else to run your illness is considerable.

Perhaps too little attention has been paid to the role of the patient in the healing process. Physicians focus on facts, not on people. So much information can be discerned from X rays, computerized scans, laboratory tests, and even Doppler, sonar, and laser technology that the patient has been displaced as the focus of the investigative process. We have entered an age where it has become increasingly common to identify and treat abnormal values, rather than to fully explore and understand the unique psychobiologic social problems of the individual.

Is there a role for the patient in the treatment of his own pain, and if so, what is it?

It is threatening to go against the grain and assume responsibility for yourself, especially in matters medical. As a society, we have conceived a generation of medical specialists so finely trained that they are thought to be able to master the explosion of technological potential that has brought a renaissance to our science. In the public's mind, the limits of knowledge are infinite. If it is specialization you seek, rest assured that there is always someone more knowledgeable to consult and counsel, someone else to inspire confidence and create hope.

Hope is fine but it will not control pain. People knowledgeable about their problems, committed to treating all aspects of their health, and willing to avoid the lure of easy cures will eventually gain mastery over their pain. In many ways, the pain-go-round is treatment without a cohesive unity of doctor and patient. It is the doctor treating the patient, not the doctor and patient aligned together treating a disease. To effectively control pain, a person must become an active participant in his health care. Frequently, it is not the treatment that fails but a lack of collaboration that undermines everyone's efforts. Use the Personal Pain Program to learn about your problem and help yourself; it may be easier than you anticipate.

Chapter 12

CONSIDERATIONS IN SELECTING A DOCTOR

HOW TO CHOOSE A COLLABORATOR

Finding the right physician can be a tough task. What are the important criteria for selecting a doctor? Must he be an internist? An orthopedic surgeon? A "pain specialist"? Is it necessary for you to like the doctor, to feel comfortable with him? How can you locate the person who is right for you?

In most cases, the person with a chronic pain problem will see more than one physician: referrals from specialist to specialist are common. Without one responsible medical leader there is a tendency to lose direction. Getting advice, consultation, medication, and treatment from a multitude of sources creates confusion. Treatment protocols can overlap and conflict. Questions arise regarding the combination of medications. The potential for drug abuse is considerable. Clearly, too many cooks can spoil the broth.

As pain is a subjective problem, the treating physician should be someone skilled in handling subjective complaints. Many doctors are not comfortable listening to patients. Some physicians are action-oriented; they want to do something for you regardless of whether or not you happen to need something done. There are physicians who do not enjoy talking about problems with patients, especially when the complaints do not deal directly with the patients' immediate treatment. These dynamics work against the collaboration process in the treatment of chronic pain. The patient may be given excellent advice, a fine choice of medication, even a plethora of appropriate medical referrals, but may wind up being inadequately monitored.

The physician may be quite efficient in making recommendations, but not very effective in establishing rapport.

The tuned-in doctor will understand the disruptive influence of chronic pain in a person's life and make comprehensive ongoing care a part of the treatment. Any treatment works best when there is an established contract, i.e., when the frequency and timing of the visits are established as part of the treatment protocol. This planning recognizes the longevity and chronicity of the problem. The patient should not be rushed into "feeling better" but encouraged to "heal" at his particular, individual rate. We have prepared a list of questions and answers that may be useful in the process of selecting a physician. If you already have a physician, try to apply some of these ideas to your present situation. Do you have a satisfactory relationship? Are you getting the most out of your physician visits?

1. **Does the doctor spend sufficient time with you to really understand your problems?**

   While there is no right amount of time to spend with a patient, you shouldn't feel rushed in your visits or as if you were imposing. Doctors are not mind readers. They do not know the details of your pain problem simply by looking at you. Good treatment depends on getting a thorough, specific history. By asking questions about your present and past health, the health problems of your family, and the details of your personal life, the doctor can get a better understanding of you as a person. Getting specific and personal information is essential. Superficial facts and generalizations add little to the understanding of a complex health problem.

2. **Does he appear interested in and concerned about your difficulties, or does he have a tendency to "dismiss" your complaints as irrelevant?**

   Patients (and we are *all*, at one time or another, patients) are often troubled by trivial and sometimes blatantly embarrassing difficulties. The doctor should seriously consider everything you tell him, for it is often the small, trivial, or minor issues that cause people the most annoyance. That is not to say that he has to sit there with a stiff upper lip and absorb everything in neutral silence. He may at times laugh and joke with you, tease you, even tell you not to worry about one thing or another. A healthy amount of personality should shine through as well as a good sense of humor. Nonetheless, the general demeanor should be one of serious deliberation; a respectful, friendly attitude will go a long way in helping to heal a sore back.

3. **Are medical tests explained? Are you aware of what will be done to you in a given procedure, and the reasons for the tests being ordered?**

All too often, patients are worked up as a matter of protocol. Simply because certain useful tests are readily available, one feels free to order them. The specificity and necessity of a test are often considered secondary to its availability and the "possibility" that it may be useful. Often, physicians perform tests because they feel compelled to do something and, not having a positive idea what to do, will order a test because that seems like the "professional" thing to do, and because it will help ease the patient's curiosity. However, before agreeing to any test or procedure, be sure the doctor knows why he is ordering it in your case. If he can explain his reasons to you, and it makes good sense (not a bunch of medical mumbo jumbo), then it would probably would be a good idea to go ahead. The rule of thumb here is that you should understand why something is being done.

Rest assured that no doctor (we've treated a number of them) would submit to any test unless he was absolutely convinced it was indicated and important. Wonder how many doctors have barium enemas as a matter of routine? Very few. Tests are serious matters when applied to oneself. A physician would not even part with an ounce of blood unnecessarily. Be fussy. Ask why, when, and even how something will be done. Do not leave anything to chance or accept the "usual procedure" nonsense.

4. **Does each new problem evoke a new round of tests? A new batch of referrals? Are tests repeated each time your problem flares? Are previous test results viewed and considered prior to ordering repeat procedures?**

Your medical records are part of your pain history. A documentation of previous treatments and test results should accompany you to each new appointment. Being sent to a new doctor without adequate referral information or available records may result in an unnecessary slew of tests and procedures. Be certain that if you go to a new doctor, he has your records. This is *your* responsibility. Ask your doctor to help you. Remind him; bug him! He is busy and he can easily overlook having your records forwarded before you. Just because a test or procedure is harmless is no reason for you to become a human guinea pig.

5. **Are referrals to other doctors followed up on adequately?**

A good primary care pain physician will not abandon you to the care of another specialist. If he feels a referral is warranted, he should explain the basis for his decision to you. A written report or phone call should precede your visit, and a follow-up report or a consultation should take place afterward. The concerned physician will follow up. He will not leave you in the lurch.

If the doctor treating you decides to transfer you to the care of another physician, as often occurs with problems of chronic pain, the reasons and rationale should be thoroughly explained. Often, certain physicians who have a special interest in treating people with chronic pain are the logical and appropriate choices to assume primary responsibility. Avoid being sent from one doctor to another simply because no one wants to assume primary responsibility. This is a fast route to the pain-go-round. Find someone who is interested in seeing you on an ongoing basis and stick with him.

6. **Can he admit he does not know? Or does he have an answer for everything?**

No one knows everything. The mind and the body are far too complex to be understood by any one person. Good medical care is not an absolute truth. It is a matter of judgment and the *best available knowledge*. Reasonableness and concern should always balance hard, cold facts. Perfection is well beyond anyone's grasp.

Humility and the expression of limited goals are often definite indications of a physician's honesty and candor. Recognizing the limits of science and operating within those boundaries are signs of competence and maturity. Beware of the doctor who has an answer or, worse yet, a pill for every ailment and complaint. There are those who profess solutions to all your aches and pains. Rest assured, it just ain't so! A wait-and-see attitude, while not immediately consoling, may prove most helpful in the long run.

7. **When a medicine or treatment is recommended, will he adequately explain the benefits, risks, and possible side effects?**

Perhaps the most difficult aspect of medicine lies in prescribing medications properly. It has been proven that a placebo—an inert medication—will provide a therapeutic benefit in over one third of the patients receiving it. This effect is a function of the patient's attitude. He believes in the efficacy of the medication. Understanding how a medication works and *wanting it to be effective* are critical elements affecting drug efficacy. This beneficial effect is dependent on the facilitatory role of the physician who conveys a positive, knowledgeable, and enthusiastic attitude about the medication.

Most medications used in chronic pain—such as analgesics, antidepressants, or sleeping medications—are potentially dangerous. They demand sound judgment in choosing them, instruction in how to use them, and due consideration of their effect. Regular office follow-up is essential. Anyone who simply gives you a prescription with either unlimited or freely available refills is not doing you a service. Stabilizing you on medication requires time and patience.

Knowing how a medication works and what side effects you may experience and understanding the potential benefits and risks will help you use the medication wisely and to best advantage.

8. **Are medications rapidly switched or changed without adequate trial or explanation?**

It may take many weeks for a particular medication to become effective. Giving up too early on a drug may deprive you of the potential therapeutic benefit. Medications often alter the body's physiological and psychological equilibrium. Allowing adequate time for equilibration may offset some adverse drug effects. Many people become unduly frightened by minor changes produced by medication. A physician who has adequately prepared his patients and can periodically reassure them offers the best opportunity for ensuring drug compliance and gaining drug benefit.

Studies done of drug compliance at medical clinics bear this out. Anywhere from 50 to 90 percent of the prescriptions written by the clinic's doctors get thrown out. That is, they do not even get filled. In one study, a trash can was strategically placed outside the clinic's door. At the end of the day, 40 percent of the prescriptions written by the clinic's doctors wound up in that can. For whatever reason, people simply had no intention of taking the medication they were prescribed.

Even filling the prescription does not ensure that the medication will be used properly. In another study, a group of social workers made regular home visits to elderly and disabled patients, many of whom suffered from chronic pain problems. Almost uniformly, these workers reported finding bottles upon bottles of medications. Typically each bottle would be missing two to five tablets. Every few months the medications would be renewed by the prescribing physician or some other physician, and a new bottle of medication would be provided by the pharmacist. Yet the skeptical, apprehensive, depressed, or simply noncompliant patient would leave the unused medication neatly stored in the medicine cabinet or on the dresser. Many stated they had so much medication that it depressed them. So they tried not to take it. Others felt that they would take the medication only when they needed it, and therefore, made conscious efforts to avoid using it, saving it for those times when they were most distressed.

Self-medication is dangerous. It can rob you of potential benefits as well as lead to abuse and dependency problems. Having an ongoing supervising physician monitor the medication is the best insurance against abuse.

9. **Do you find that the doctor will give you anything you want—often just to appease you or keep you out of his hair?**

A sound physician does not let the patient prescribe. That is not to say that he won't listen to you, but he will not necessarily agree with you and give you anything you want. Standing up to a patient's demands, not being bullied or forced into prescribing unnecessary medication or tests, is a genuine sign of concern and competence. Sometimes people can get very angry. Being able to tolerate a patient's anger without feeling guilty, defensive, or inadequate is a difficult aspect of doctoring. Putting people off by agreeing or prescribing without sound therapeutic basis is a cop-out—a way of getting the patient off your back without really addressing his problem. Find a doctor who will stand up to you and argue reasonably and intelligently, not simply go along with whatever idea you happened to bring to the office that week. Someone who has definite opinions and will stand up for what he or she believes in will be a stabilizing factor to help you through the vicissitudes of a chronic pain syndrome.

There is no one perfect primary care doctor. But someone with a good general interest in you and your problems, someone who does not put you on the defensive, making you apologize or explain why you are still feeling poorly, will be a good choice. Find a doctor who will be patient with you. If he accepts you and recognizes the reality of your problems, he will be an excellent collaborator in the battle to control chronic pain.

HOW DOES THE "PAIN SPECIALIST" LOOK AT THE PATIENT WITH PAIN?

We use the term "pain specialist" quite pragmatically. There really is no medical specialty that authorizes physicians to hang out the shingle "pain specialist." The term is used to refer to any medical specialist who has an interest in treating patients with chronic pain. By training, that doctor may be an internist, general practitioner, family practice specialist, orthopedic surgeon, anesthesiologist, neurologist, psychiatrist, or physiatrist; virtually any medical doctor can wind up being a pain specialist. What unifies all these specialists is a certain approach to the patient, an approach that addresses all the significant aspects of his physical health, emotional well-being, and social situation. The following case history illustrates the process of holistic evaluation:

At the age of thirty-six, Tom Blake spoke of retiring.
"What would you do with yourself?" we questioned.
"Sell the house, move the family to Florida. It's hard for me to get around up here, especially when the weather is poor."
"Yes, but what will you do?" we persisted.
"What can I do? I certainly can't go back to the market. I can't lift anything. Besides, it's cheaper for them to keep me on disability than put me back on the payroll."

Tom Blake had given up. He was retiring not only from his job but from life. In order to promote any positive charge, we felt we had to address his defeatism.

"Do you mean that at your age there is nothing more you want to do, that you will be content to go to Florida and sit in the sun, fish, play golf, for the rest of your life?"
"As long as I get workmen's compensation, social security dis-

ability, I will be financially set for the rest of my life. Of course I'm not happy with that, but what else can I do?"

Tom had been the assistant manager of a large store in Washington, D.C., prior to sustaining a back injury. After the injury, he returned to work despite some vague, nagging discomfort in his back. Four months later, his mother died suddenly from a heart attack. Although he was quite close to his mother, her death was quickly mourned, and after a brief absence he again returned to work. But nothing was the same.

Depression ensued. His enthusiasm waned. He spent more time sitting around the house. The vague pain in his back became a more severe pain, a constant irritant curtailing his activities and limiting his capacity to work. The pain cycle had started.

He sought medical consultation a full six months after the original injury and two months following his mother's death. His family physician, after listening attentively to details of the original fall and the persistent discomfort, diagnosed lumbar strain. He advised a week of bed rest and some adjunctive aspirin and Valium. The subsequent week in bed, while successfully resting the inflammation in his back, exacerbated Tom's depressed feelings by forcing him to focus on his poor aching back and not the details of his responsibilities at work. The failure of "conservative treatment" necessitated an orthopedic referral.

Tom's X rays were normal and physical examination did not reveal neurological damage. The pain persisted; the surgeon requested that he return in one month if he did not improve.

Conditions at work demanded his immediate return. An inventory-control system he had created required reevaluation and his expertise was required. He had to go back despite the fact that he was not feeling well. The orthopedic surgeon prescribed large doses of aspirin and muscle relaxants to reduce some of the spasms. He was well medicated, if not a bit sedated. Whereas previously he would have spent whatever time was necessary to seek the source of the difficulty at work and implement a solution (qualities of persistence and dedication that had contributed to his rapid promotion within the organization), he found that he now lacked motivation. His back hurt and compromised his concentration. The combination of Valium and aspirin gave rise to episodic nausea and unpredictable bouts of drowsiness. The burden of work became overwhelming. Although he continued to drag himself to work each day, he dreaded

waking up in the morning. Twelve days after returning to work he
called in sick. In his head, he knew that he was not really sick, at
least no sicker than he was the day before when he had worked.
Tom rationalized. Instead of pushing himself through another day,
he would rest, allow himself to regain his full effectiveness. It was
the first time in his life he had allowed himself to call in sick when
he knew in his heart he really could have made it. For Tom this was
the turning point.

Chronic pain had begun to erode Tom's confidence. He was no
longer the same person. Not because Tom was weak; quite the contrary. He was a very strong willed, self-determined man who in the
course of his life had proven the strength of his character to everyone who knew him. He now had a chronic pain syndrome and the
pervasive, destructive power of that condition was invading his life
space.

Let us examine his pain system profile:

Tom Blake's Pain System Profile

IDENTIFYING INFORMATION: BLAKE, THOMAS (36)
   Assistant manager, Free House Corporation
   Married (14 years)
   Three daughters (12, 10, 6)
   Diagnosis: Chronic pain syndrome
                Chronic lumbosacral strain
   Currently receiving workmen's compensation, Social Security Dis-
      ability
ASSETS: Intelligent, hard worker, determined, persistent nature
LIABILITIES:
   Overly sensitive to criticism
   Has tendency to be stubborn
   Domineering, tends to be very self-directed, especially when under
      stress
   Fiercely independent to the point of not asking for help, especially
      when needed
FAMILY: Type III family has been so subjugated by Tom that in
   the absence of his leadership seems lost and confused about what
   to do for him
MAJOR PHYSICAL PROBLEMS:
   1. mild hypertensive cardiovascular disease

2. recurrent severe lumbosacral strain

FITNESS:

1. Mild obesity (25 pounds overweight)
2. Poor exercise tolerance
3. Absence of appropriate conditioning program

HABITS:

1. Cigarettes—1½ packs per day
2. Tendency, under stress, to drink too much

MEDICATION:

1. Aspirin (10 tablets per day)
   Complications: persistent epigastritis, preulcer pathology, minimal pain control
2. Valium (25 mg daily)
   Complications: drowsiness, diminished concentration, fatigue, early onset of tranquilizer-induced depression

PERSONALITY CHANGES DURING COURSE OF ILLNESS:

1. *Loss of confidence* in his ability to work effectively
2. *Rationalization* that his injury and pain will get better with complete rest. *Denial* of poor physical condition and chronic medication problems.
3. Major change in relationship with family, who have lost his leadership and are *helpless* to provide direction.
4. With loss of daily job routine and structure, he experiences *negative self-worth feedback,* which increases depression.

PREDICTED COURSE:

1. With each day out of work, moves further away from ever returning to former level of job performance.
2. Continuation of family floundering, with members eventually moving in independent, self-serving directions.
3. Continuation of drug(Valium)-induced depressive illness.
4. With continued aspirin use, the development of gastric ulceration.

The profile is a summary of what might appear in the physician's chart. It first assesses all the positive and negative factors that affect a person's pain. Then, the type of treatment he is currently receiving is specified, and from the data, a course of recovery is predicted. It may be useful for you to sit down, and using Tom Blake's form as a model, begin to outline your own pain profile. It might give you some interesting facts upon which to base future treatment decisions.

Chapter 13

MEDICINES FOR PAIN

THE "THERAPEUTIC JUNGLE"

In 1954, Drs. Louis Goodman and Alfred Gilman reauthored a textbook that has become a medical classic, *The Pharmacological Basis of Therapeutics*. They wrote the original text in 1940 as a guide for physicians and medical students in the judicious use of drugs in medicine. By 1954, the world had changed. As the doctors noted, "In a real sense, this second edition constitutes a complete revision of the first edition. The 14 years that have separated the two books have witnessed pharmacological and therapeutic advances which are probably unparalleled in the history of medicine."

Of particular interest was the addition of a new objective to this second edition, ". . . namely, to provide the reader with a way of thinking about drugs" so that he will be better prepared to withstand the flood of unsubstantiated claims that are often made for new drugs, and to evaluate critically the published literature on the properties and uses of the many new therapeutic agents in comparison to the older, well-established compounds of the same class.

By the time the third edition was written in 1966, the authors had become editors, no longer able to personally document and organize the magnitude of new information in the field of medical pharmacology. A project that began in 1940 as the work of two men became a massive compendium of forty-two collaborators. As a consequence of this accidental growth and knowledge, the editors warned that "parallel with important advances in the basic medical disciplines, there has been an ever increasing number of new drugs available to the physician and a thickening of what has become the therapeutic jungle."

All that is new is not necessarily better. Often change represents inconsequential or meaningless differences. The physician as consumer, dispenser of prescriptions, has become the marketing object of a multibillion-dollar drug industry. How does one find one's way in the therapeutic jungle? Do multicolor ads, free audio cassettes, and a closetful of physician's samples help one choose from a marketplace flooded with the questionable promise of invention, innovation, and improvement?

The choice of therapy is really more limited than we would like our patients to believe. The basics are still the basics. For example, the use of aspirin, a well-established "old" remedy is still, in 1981, the mainstay of treatment for chronic pain.

The proven and trusted methods of drug treatment persist because they are effective and useful. While considerable progress in drug research has brought improvement in many areas, the advances in the pharmacological treatment of pain have been slow and tedious. While many claims are made for new and better remedies, genuine advances are few and far between. Progress in medical therapeutics is always precarious, for the solutions to any one problem are not absolute but must be considered with due regard for their effect on the entire human system. The balance of benefit vs. risk is at the heart of the therapeutic dilemma. The choice is often difficult, the pressure to try something new is omnipresent.

Drs. Goodman and Gilman provided sage advice for the physician in the preface to the third edition of their text, and their comments are equally important for patients as well: ". . . in the area where the number of therapeutic agents available is exceedingly large . . . the physician is advised not to be the first to adopt the new remedy nor the last to discard the old."

NOT TO BE UNDERESTIMATED: MEDICINE TRIED AND TRUE

It's 8 P.M. You have dragged yourself through a torturous day at the office. Wading through the traffic home was abysmal, dinner was overdone, and by the time you have gotten the children to bed your head is about to fall off. Your favorite television program has been canceled and in its place is the story of two single women living alone in New York City trying to find work doing soap operas. The show stinks, you are getting nauseated.

As the action breaks, a word from our sponsors brings us a man in a white coat studiously poised over two identical Erlenmeyer flasks. He pours a white powder into each flask and stirs the solution with a glass rod. Confidently, the professor examines both flasks, adjusts his bifocals, and cryptically comments, "Solution A has more of the ingredient most effective in the relief of pain and clearly goes to work faster." Miracles exist! Especially if you decide to have your stomach replaced with an Erlenmeyer flask.

What they are advertising is no magic, but an ancient remedy for fevers. First discovered by the Greeks, willow bark (salix alba) was the ancient source of salicin. Chemical analysis in the nineteenth century produced a compound that yielded salicylic acid and ultimately acetylsalicylic acid, or aspirin—the ultimate pain reliever.

Aspirin is a remarkable drug in the treatment of pain. Although the drug has been around for hundreds of years, researchers are still finding new and previously unknown mechanisms by which it affects the human body. Most recently, its anticoagulant effects have been discovered, making aspirin a safe, low-cost agent for thinning the blood. Traditionally, aspirin has been accepted to have three major therapeutic actions:

1. *Antipyresis* (*lowering the body temperature*). Aspirin will act to lower the body temperature in a rapid and effective manner in those conditions where the temperature is abnormally high. It will not lower the body temperature itself. Instead, it acts by resetting the temperature-regulating mechanism in the brain.

2. *Analgesia* (*alleviation of pain*). Although the mechanism by which aspirin alleviates pain is not yet fully understood, it is thought to act by a selective depressant effect on the central nervous system. Aspirin dulls the brain's awareness of pain.

3. *Anti-inflammatory effect* (*reduction of swelling at the site of injury*). A portion of the pain-relieving function of aspirin is due to an effect at the site of injury, a prevention and alleviation of the inflammation and a consequent removal of one source of stimulation of the pain receptors.

The three-faceted effect of aspirin, its relative safety even in moderately high doses, and the general effectiveness of the drug in the control and treatment of mild to moderate pain all contribute to its longevity and popularity as a pain reliever. Salicylates seem to be effective for pain of low intensity, whether the pain is localized to (headache) or widespread (generalized muscle pain), and pain that arises from the muscles, bones, and ligaments as opposed to pain from organs.

Aspirin and Its Many Combinations

The limitation with aspirin is clearly its low threshold: it is much more effective with low-intensity pain than with severe pain. Hence, aspirin is frequently combined with other analgesics and sedatives in "combination" preparations designed to provide more effective pain relief than can be obtained with any one of the agents alone.

ASCRIPTIN*

This drug combines aspirin with Maalox* (magnesium-aluminum hydroxide), a potent antacid.

Rationale:

Aspirin is extremely irritating to the stomach and intestines. Some reports, in fact, indicate that as little as one dose of aspirin can produce stomach bleeding. The very small amount of bleeding that may occur with aspirin is painless, unless the aspirin actually erodes the intestinal lining, producing an ulcer, which is very painful. Otherwise, the bleeding from aspirin goes largely unnoticed, leading to blood loss in the stool or occasionally to iron-deficiency anemia. In most cases where aspirin is used, moderate bleeding is not significant.

To prevent bleeding or gastric irritation (symptoms of heartburn, indigestion, stomach discomfort), aspirin is best taken on a full stomach or with food. Another method for minimizing the erosive effect is to combine the aspirin with a buffering compound. Ascriptin is an example of such a product. Maalox acts to neutralize the gastric acid and increase the tolerance to aspirin.

Indication:

A wide range of conditions where aspirin is the drug of choice (mild to moderate pain, especially from the muscles, bones, and joints). The buffering capacity of this medication makes it particularly useful in arthritis and other chronic pain conditions where the long-term use of aspirin is indicated.

Warning:

1. Aspirin is toxic in sufficiently high doses. It can cause confu-

* Asterisks denote brand names.

sion, dizziness, gastric irritation, and ringing in the ears when present in excessive amounts.

Comments:

Aspirin is the mainstay of treatment of chronic pain of mild to moderate severity. Ascriptin or buffered aspirin is generally better tolerated, especially over the longer term. Despite the presence of antacids, aspirin is still a potent irritant and may produce a full range of gastric symptoms. While buffered preparations may help certain individuals, they are not certain protection against bleeding and ulcer. Combination drugs strive to maximize the analgesic effect of aspirin by combining it with other pain-relieving medications. The following list describes the more common preparations:

FIORINAL*

This drug combines aspirin with phenacetin and caffeine and adds a short- to medium-term barbiturate. (Short-term is under two hours; medium is up to four hours; long-acting is eight to twelve hours.)

Rationale:

The drug is specifically formulated for the treatment of headache pain, or psychic tension and muscle contraction in the head, neck, and shoulder regions. The addition of a barbiturate adds a sedating effect to the analgesic of aspirin. The drug is extremely popular, substantiating the apparent effectiveness of the medication in the treatment of headache, especially in the acute phase and over the brief term (and substantiating as well, perhaps, the effectiveness of some rather aggressive marketing of the product).

Indications:

For relief of the symptom complex of tension (muscle contraction) headache.

Major Warning:
1. *Drug dependency.* The prolonged use of barbiturates can easily produce both psychic and physical dependence. As tension headache symptoms are by nature long-term illnesses, the potential for drug abuse and dependency exists.
2. *Barbiturates* act by depressing the central nervous system. Barbiturates can dull mental alertness and hamper the performance of potentially hazardous tasks.

Comments:

Fiorinal can be used in the acute phases of tension headache. The regular continued use of the drug is likely to result in dependency or abuse. The drug is also available as Fiorinal with codeine, which may contain either one eighth, one quarter, or one half grain of codeine phosphate.

EQUAGESIC*

This is a combination of aspirin with meprobamate (a tranquilizer, Miltown*) and ethoheptazine citrate (an analgesic whose mechanism of action is not proven).

Rationale:

The combination of meprobamate, a drug commonly used in the treatment of tension and anxiety, with two other analgesic agents is designed to produce a summation effect. The implication is that anxiety and tension play a role in exacerbating and perpetuating the pain.

Indications:

Basing its findings on a review of this drug by the National Academy of Science / National Research Council, and other information, the FDA has classified the indications as follows: "Possibly effective: for the treatment of pain accompanied by tension and/or anxiety in patients with musculoskelctal disorders or tension headaches."

The effectiveness of Equagesic in long-term use—that is, more than four months—has not been assessed by systematic clinical studies. The FDA warns, "Physicians should periodically reassess the usefulness of the drug for individual patients."

Warnings:

1. Meprobamate has a propensity to produce drug dependency.
2. Rapid withdrawal of the drug, particularly after prolonged usage, can result in a withdrawal syndrome, including psychological excitement, confusion, agitation, and possibly seizure.

Comment:

The combination of potentially addictive tranquilizers with aspirin is problematic in the chronic pain condition. Aspirin is a long-term treatment for chronic pain; tranquilizers, especially the potentially addictive ones, are appropriate only in moderate doses for brief periods: they are a short-term measure. Combining a long-term mainstay such as aspirin with a tranquilizer can often lead to someone who needs the aspirin taking too much of the tranquilizer. Short-term, limited use of this drug may prove useful when pain and anxiety are manifest; however, combining these agents makes little sense for long-term pain management.

Nonnarcotic Analgesics—Newer than Aspirin

Several new compounds have been introduced in recent years that are useful in alleviating mild to moderately severe pain and are useful in both long- and short-term problems. All of this is without the potential for addiction. There are a number of newer drugs with pain relieving and anti-inflammatory properties that merit discussion:

ZOMAX* (zomepirac sodium)

This drug is a nonsteroidal, anti-inflammatory agent which has been developed as an analgesic. It can also lower fever (antipyretic property).

It is not entirely clear how this drug works in relieving pain, but it is theorized that it inhibits the synthesis of certain circulating substances in the body called prostaglandins. Recent research has indicated that prostaglandins are present in various pain-producing conditions; for example, they produce contractions of the uterus, causing menstrual cramps, and can constrict smooth muscle resulting in headaches. Inhibiting their synthesis with medications like Zomax may play an important role in pain relief.

Indications:

This medication is indicated in both acute and chronic pain conditions. In a study of patients with chronic orthopedic pain due to degenerative joint disease, 85 percent found the drug helpful in the management of their pain.

Warnings:

1. The most frequent complication reported in the initial trials with this drug are gastrointestinal complaints, specifically nausea (12 percent).
2. The incidence of vomiting, constipation, stomach pain, diarrhea, indigestion, dizziness, insomnia, edema (swelling of the ankles or hands), high blood pressure, and rash were reported in anywhere from 3 to 9 percent of the patients taking the drug.
3. Certain changes in kidney function have been reported with the

long-term use of this drug in monkeys. Therefore, humans using the drug over a period of months should have their renal function periodically tested.

Comments:

The concept of an analgesic that can effectively reduce pain by inhibiting the body's synthesis of pain-producing compounds is extremely promising. As the drug is new, the benefit in the long-term management of pain remains to be proven. It should be noted, however, that the incidence of moderately unpleasant side effects is relatively high.

MOTRIN* (ibuprofen)

This is an anti-inflammatory agent that possesses analgesic and antipyretic activity.

This drug has been widely used in the treatment of rheumatoid arthritis and osteoarthritis. The drug is reported to reduce pain and decrease the severity of morning stiffness, as well as increase the strength of the handicapped arthritic, increase mobility, and delay the onset of fatigue.

Originally thought to exert its pain relief by virtue of anti-inflammatory action, the drug is currently thought to possess a capacity to inhibit prostaglandin synthesis.

Indications:

It is indicated for the signs and symptoms of rheumatoid arthritis and osteoarthritis. It can be used to control acute flare-ups as well as play a part in the long-term management of these diseases.

Warnings:

1. This drug is particularly irritating to the stomach and intestines. In some studies as many as 16 percent of those using the medication have reported gastrointestinal side effects.
2. The drug may produce blurred or diminished vision. This side effect may be transitory, but should signal prompt discontinuation of the drug.
3. The drug should not be given to individuals who are also on blood thinners (Coumadin*-type).

Comments:

Motrin and other similar compounds have been very helpful in the treatment of arthritis. Recently they have been used to treat menstrual cramps. This medication has been very popular among pain patients generally and especially those with severe arthritis. The gastrointestinal effects have made taking the drug regularly over the long term rather difficult for many people.

CLINORIL* (fulindac) and others

This medication has only recently been available in the United States for the treatment of arthritic disorders. It has received a great deal of favorable press and media attention resulting in a broad public awareness. Many pain patients have requested their physicians to prescribe it.

Like the nonsteroidal anti-inflammatory drugs, such as Nalfon,* Naprosyn,* Tolectin,* and Anaprox,* Clinoril inhibits prostaglandin synthesis and thus reduces inflammation and alleviates pain. The studies that compared Clinoril with Motrin and aspirin found that in patients with rheumatoid arthritis, Clinoril in doses of 300–400 mg daily was as effective as 3600 mg to 4800 mg of aspirin per day, and in osteoarthritis of the hip or knee it was as effective as 3600 mg aspirin per day.

Most studies have shown that all the nonsteroidal anti-inflammatory drugs are basically equally effective in the short-term treatment of the arthritic disorders. As most types of arthritis and many of the chronic pain syndromes require treatment over many years, the safety and long-term effectiveness of these drugs remain to be proven. As to which drugs to choose, the decision should be left to your physician. These are potent drugs and their clinical usefulness may be more limited than their press and media hype seems to indicate. They are not for everyone. Nonetheless, if you are given a trial of one of these compounds, be sure to carefully monitor the benefits and side effects. Certain people seem to do better and have fewer side effects on a particular drug. A bit of experimentation is often the only way to find what works best for you.

As a general rule, most of these compounds are best tolerated if taken with food to minimize gastric irritation. Despite manufacturers' claims, none is really well tolerated on a long-term basis. Careful collaboration with your physician will minimize problems. We feel that conscientious use of the pain diary medication record will be extremely helpful in obtaining the maximum therapeutic benefit.

Narcotics—Potential for Abuse

Narcotics are drugs that relieve pain and produce sleep. Morphine is the standard against which all other narcotic analgesics are measured. All narcotic agents are addicting, producing physical as well as psychological addiction. Although many nonaddicting synthetics, adequate for managing mild to moderate pain, have been produced, none are adequate to manage severe pain.

As chronic pain states are long-term conditions, the utility of narcotics in the management of these states is extremely limited: the potential for dependency and abuse is simply too high. This is not to imply that narcotics are not prescribed; they are frequently thought to be a good short-term means of controlling pain. Rarely do the benign pain states benefit from narcotic intervention.

It is thought that opium was first used even before history was recorded. The word "opium" comes from the Greek name for juice, the drug being obtained from the juice of the poppy capsules.

Opium was widely introduced throughout the world. By the middle of the sixteenth century the analgesic use of opium was fairly common in Europe. In 1803, a young German pharmacist named Sertürner isolated morphine from opium and named the drug after Morpheus, the Greek god of dreams.

The availability of morphine revolutionized the use of opiates. With the invention of the hypodermic needle, the ability to inject pure refined morphine directly into the blood system produced the potential for severe addiction. The relatively easy availability of the drug, the profound euphoric effect of direct injection, and the enormous addictive property of the drug created an epidemic of opiate addiction that has persisted to the present time.

THE PROPERTIES OF MORPHINE

In all the history of the world there is no more potent and pain-relieving substance than morphine. It has been smoked, swallowed, and injected to alter consciousness. In addition to relieving pain, the drug produces drowsiness, changes moods, and creates mental clouding. In the process of removing pain and discomfort, worry and tension, it can create euphoria.

Morphine can relieve pain in a selective manner, without diminishing the sense perception of touch, vibration, vision, hearing, etc. In fact, even the perception of pain itself is not altered. People still perceive pain, but the reaction to the pain is altered; morphine affects only the reaction to pain and not the original sensation of pain. A subject receiving morphine can recognize the sensation of pain but is comfortable with the pain.

One possible interpretation of this effect is the ability of morphine to divest pain of its capacity to evoke its usual responses—anxiety, anticipation, fear, and suffering—the series of responses that fuel the pain-go-round. The reaction to morphine is quite variable.

WHAT IS DRUG DEPENDENCE?

"Nothing is more desirable than to be released from affliction, but nothing is more frightening than to be divested of a crutch."

JAMES BALDWIN, *Nobody Knows My Name*

No one likes to think that he or she has a drug problem. Drug dependency is a touchy subject. The vast majority of people we questioned denied needing continued medication. If the results of a study conducted at the Mayo Clinic in 1979 are applicable to the general population, then the extent of the problem is enormous. Of 144 patients with chronic pain of nonmalignancy cause, 35 (24 percent) were drug-dependent, 59 (41 percent) drug abusers, and 50 (35 percent) nonabusers.

Fully two thirds of all chronic pain patients were either dependent or abusers. The study group provided the following definition of drug dependency:

No medical explanation for the sustained use of a drug, and one of the following:

1. The increasing daily dose of a narcotic for more than a month (ultimately *exceeding* the recommended maximum dose).
2. Simultaneous use of two kinds of narcotics.
3. Increasing daily doses of nonnarcotic drugs for more than a month (ultimately exceeding twice the recommended maximum dose).

Drug abuse was defined as:

No medical evidence to warrant the sustained use of a drug, and one of the following:

1. Exceeding the daily recommended dosage of narcotic pain medication for more than one month.
2. The use of nonnarcotic pain medication exceeding the daily recommended dosage on a daily basis for more than a month.
3. The simultaneous use of four or more pain medications on a daily basis for more than a month.

What Drugs Are Most Commonly Abused?

The Mayo Clinic study reveals that codeine and oxycodone (Percodan*) were the drugs most likely to be abused. Sixty percent of the drug abusers and 75 percent of the drug-dependent patients were misusing one of these two drugs.

The reason for the widespread abuse of codeine is its ubiquitous presence in combination pain medication. It is present in forty-two different combination drugs. It is no wonder that many of the patients in the Mayo Clinic study didn't even realize they were taking the drug. The study group found that "regardless of whether they were physically dependent or not, oxycodone (Percodan) abusers had difficulty in stopping their medication." The high addictive risk associated with the use of Percodan has also been confirmed by our clinical experience with patients. While these two agents stand out as major elements of abuse, any narcotic or nonnarcotic agent is potentially dangerous, especially in the treatment of chronic, unremitting pain. If you meet the criteria of drug abuse or dependency, consult your physician. Telling someone is the first step to getting unhooked.

Why People Get Hooked on Drugs

Many individuals will "explain" their use of drugs by contending they are the involuntary victims of their pain. Receiving narcotics prescriptions, often from more than one doctor, creates availability. Having the drugs accessible enhances the likelihood of their potential abuse. The following case history highlights the dilemma of accessibility:

Joanne was a twenty-nine-year-old woman who for many years experienced severe menstrual irregularity with cramping and pain. During her twenties she simply tolerated the monthly discomfort as best she could, missing a few days of work once or twice a year. At age twenty-seven she had occasion to change gynecologists and was advised to use a combination of Naprosyn and Tylenol ℀3* with codeine for her cramps. She found the codeine upset her stomach but reduced the severity of her cramps.

Two years later she pulled out her back doing some heavy lifting in the office. She saw an orthopedic surgeon who started her on Percodan and a muscle relaxant. She found the Percodan really put her "out of touch," a feeling that she was unaccustomed to but sort of liked. She began to forget what she was taking and started to pop pills fairly regularly—that is, until she ran out of medication. Then she simply called the doctor's office and had her prescription renewed; the ease of procurement surprised her.

As time passed she found she was using more of the Percodan to provide a given amount of pain relief. In fact, she would run through a month's prescription in about ten days.

She made an appointment to see the orthopedic surgeon to complain about the persistent pain. He confronted her on the use of Percodan and suggested she voluntarily discontinue the drug.

A second opinion was sought. The consultant recommended hospitalization and traction. She refused and requested medication for pain relief, stating her need to continue working. The doctor reluctantly accepted her decision and prescribed Tylenol #3 with codeine. Joanne was again surprised by the ease of obtaining a narcotic prescription.

As it only took a few days to run through a month's supply of narcotics, she was forced to continually seek new sources of supply. Her tolerance for the medication was astonishing. Fortunately, her medical insurance reimbursed a major portion of her consultation fees as well as the cost of the drugs. Over the course of the next twelve months, she saw seventeen different physicians and received seventy-six different narcotic prescriptions.

Eventually, Joanne could no longer tolerate the stress of her profound drug addiction. Her back pain continued to torment her despite her ingestion of enormous doses of medication. She collapsed one evening at home, was taken by the Rescue Squad to the local hospital, and subsequently transferred to a drug detoxification center.

Chronic pain clearly predisposes one to develop a drug dependency or abuse problem. Some substances, particularly the narcotic pain relievers that alter mood, relieve tension, and produce euphoria, are more likely to be used compulsively than others; that is, they have a higher abuse liability. In addition, the narcotics are associated with a high propensity to produce tolerance—a condition where an increased amount of drug is required to produce a specific constant drug effect.

GUIDELINES FOR THE USE OF NARCOTIC AGENTS

The value of narcotics in the long-term treatment of chronic pain is doubtful. The potential for the development of tolerance and eventual drug abuse far outweigh any potential benefit in terms of analgesia. We see a role for these agents as temporary stopgap measures to relieve sudden dramatic exacerbations of a pain syndrome. In these cases the drugs should be used *exactly* as prescribed by the attending physician. Increasing the dose, exceeding maximum dose, or prolonging therapy beyond the prescribed time period is dangerous.

OTHER DRUGS IN THE TREATMENT OF PAIN

MUSCLE RELAXANTS

One of the more common causes of chronic pain is persistent muscle contraction. Physicians frequently prescribe specific muscle relaxants for the short-term management of skeletal muscle spasm. Paraflex* (chlorzoxazone), Robaxan* (methocarbamol), and Flexeril* (cyclobenzaprine) are three of the more common muscle relaxants. The drug companies propose rather sophisticated mechanisms of action for these medications. They claim that they act on the central nervous system by affecting the nerves controlling the muscles which are in spasm. A bombardment of nerve impulses throws the muscles into taut contractions (a state of overcontraction, like a clock spring wound too tightly to release itself) and produces a pain state. Muscle spasm is a major contributor to chronic pain.

In many clinical trials these drugs are found to be moderately effective in lessening spasm and the resultant pain. They seem to be relatively safe; for example, according to the drug literature on Paraflex and other compounds containing the muscle relaxant chlorzoxazone, chlorzoxazone "has been used in over 20 million patients and has been found to be well tolerated and seldom produces undesirable side effects." The usual problems include gastrointestinal irritation, drowsiness, dizziness, light-headedness, and occasional rashes—all minor annoyances as opposed to serious complications.

In our experience, muscle relaxants are a valuable adjunct to rest, appropriate conditioning, applied heat, and physical therapy in the treatment of acute painful muscle spasm. According to the FDA, the mode of action of these drugs has not been clearly determined but may be related to their sedative properties, not to their ability to relax tense muscles. In this regard we have found that small doses of the minor tranquilizer Valium* (diazepam) can be as effective in promoting muscle relaxation and the relief of spasm as any muscle relaxant. Remember, Valium is potentially dangerous if used excessively or for prolonged periods, especially without appropriate supervision.

ANTIDEPRESSANTS

Physicians are becoming increasingly aware of the utility of antidepressant medication in the long-term management of the pain states. Depression is a constant companion of pain, often creating definite biological changes in the human system that sensitize the body to pain.

The symptoms of depression—fatigue, irritability, insomnia, agitation—all intensify the experience of pain. While the neurochemical mechanism for this effect is not well known, studies have shown that depression is associated with a depletion of essential brain chemicals (catecholamines and feratonin) that are responsible for creating a sense of well-being. Since depression and chronic pain go hand in hand, treating one without the other is futile. There is literature documenting the usefulness of antidepressant medication when treating chronic musculoskeletal pain, tension and vascular headache, and pain of nonspecific origin.

There are two broad types of antidepressants currently available: the *tricyclics* and the *monoamine oxidase inhibitors*. The tricyclics are by far the more commonly prescribed. Elavil* (amitriptyline), a very popular tricyclic, can produce drowsiness, a dry mouth, and light-headedness, side effects that can easily discourage the poorly supervised or unmotivated patient. While antidepressant therapy can be effective in managing pain and diminishing the need for high doses of analgesics, it is critical to give the medication in a sufficient dose over an extended period to ensure maximum benefit. These drugs work best under the careful supervision of a trained physician familiar with their use, and when accompanied by either supportive counseling or therapy.

SPECIAL DRUGS FOR SPECIAL CONDITIONS

Two drugs, Tegretol* and Dilantin,* deserve special mention, for they play a part in special conditions. The most common use for Dilantin and Tegretol is in the treatment of epilepsy, where they are used to prevent the discharge of electrical impulses when they are not wanted, such as in the start of an epileptic seizure. It was found several years ago that these drugs can also be helpful in those conditions where peripheral nerves—that is, nerves outside the brain—are firing uncontrollably. The condition called tic douloureux, a painful facial neuritis, has been successfully treated with the drug Tegretol. In addition, those syndromes characterized by a neuritic type of pain, that is, sharp, burning, or boring pain caused by direct involvement of a nerve, are susceptible very often to the quenching effect of Dilantin and Tegretol. Peripheral neuromas (small balls at the end of nerves that have been cut during surgery) are included in this group. It is important to note, however, that the levels of Tegretol and Dilantin must be monitored carefully. This can be done by a blood test. There are significant complications that can occur with long-term use of Tegretol and Dilantin. When properly monitored, however, they serve a very useful purpose.

One further syndrome to mention is post-herpetic neuralgia. This neuralgia occurs after the disease called shingles has abated. Shingles is caused by the virus herpes zoster. (There is some thought that shingles may be the reactivation of a latent varicella virus, which is the same virus that causes chicken pox in children.) The viral infection occurs along the pathways of peripheral nerves, leaving a band or strip of pain that follows the course of the nerve. To treat post-herpetic neuralgia, one may use a combination drug regimen of an antidepressant and a major tranquilizer (often a phenothiazine). The success of this therapy has prompted doctors to use this drug combination for many other pain syndromes, in most cases with only limited success.

NEW DRUGS

There are several new drugs on the market, many of which have had adequate trials. These include Buprenorphine,* a potent narcotic analgesic that is many times more potent than morphine and that seems to be of use in cancer patients with intractable pain. The drug Butorphenol tartrate, a new analgesic chemically related to morphine, was recently approved by the FDA after clinical studies on more than four thousand patients. It seems to be an effective analgesic for moderate to severe pain, and it is twenty to forty times more potent than morphine. Several studies of this oral medication in postoperative pain show that lower amounts of Butorphenol* are analgesically equivalent to over 60 milligrams of codeine and much superior to many other kinds of analgesics.

A special word on the compound dimethylsulfoxide, or DMSO. This seems to be the newest fad drug in the treatment of pain. It has been around for many years and has been used as a solvent and a pain-killer for horses. It is a potent solvent and it penetrates the skin rapidly. A drop of DMSO on the skin can be perceived thirteen seconds later as a garlicky taste in the mouth, indicating that it has been absorbed into the bloodstream and has reached the taste buds. There are some people who claim that DMSO is an effective analgesic. There are clinics in some states which use DMSO exclusively, either by injection or by topical application. The use of DMSO is illegal in most states. Our recommendation for the use of DMSO is simple: don't. Many clinical studies done with DMSO so far are unscientific, and there is no documented proof—only anecdotal reports —that it has helped pain. It carries with it the risks of reducing the clotting mechanism in blood to dangerous levels. We recommend that you wait for the FDA to thoroughly assess this drug's clinical efficacy and safety before you attempt to use it.

Are You Using Your Medication Correctly?

There are numerous factors that *greatly* influence the effect of drugs. Simply being prescribed the correct drug and then swallowing the pill is no assurance that you will derive the intended benefit. The following are some of the more important factors that influence the effect of the drug:

THE GENETIC VARIATION BETWEEN PEOPLE

The thrust of our entire approach to pain has been to accentuate the differences among people and the need to individualize any treatment approach. The variability of response is particularly true in the area of drugs. Genetic factors are extremely important in determining the quantitative and qualitative activity of a drug. The rate at which a drug is metabolized (inactivated), the susceptibility of certain cells to the toxic effects of drugs, and the rate at which drugs are transferred around the body are all, to some degree, influenced by individual's unique genetic engineering.

AGE AND THE AMOUNT OF MEDICATION

Very young and very old people are particularly sensitive to drug effects. The young have immature metabolic and excretory systems; they cannot inactivate medications and excrete them from their bodies as rapidly as adults, and therefore they are often exquisitely sensitive to even small doses of medication.

The typical burdens of the elderly—physical impairment, decreased metabolic rate, concomitant physical illnesses, and the simultaneous use of alternate drugs—all sensitize them to particular drugs. This extreme sensitivity necessitates numerous precautions in drug prescriptions. We always start elderly patients at the lowest possible dosage of a medication, carefully observe the effect over a time, and then, only gradually and in minute increments, increase the dosage. Toxic levels are frequently encountered at quite minimal dosages. Frequently, the toxic level is reached before therapeutic benefit is achieved, rendering any potential benefits superfluous.

While dosage variations are obvious at extremes of the age spectrum, considerable variations exist among all adults as a function of how rapidly they age. Again, individual tailoring is a real necessity.

BODY WEIGHT

The size and composition of your body plays an enormous role in the amount and distribution of drugs in the body. The recommended dosages of most medications are initially formulated on a basis of drug per unit of body weight. Extreme obesity can affect "drug distribution" in the body as many drugs are lipid-loving and exhibit a predilection for attaching themselves to fat cells. The result is that certain drugs tend to build up in the fat cells of the body and not in the tissues and organs where they would be pharmacologically effective. Individuals with little body fat may experience an "overdose" effect, as little of the ingested drug is bound up in fat and the whole bolus of the drug goes to work at once.

SEX AND PILLS

Despite the need for greater equality under the law, physiological systems remain biologically prejudicial. In general, women are thought to be more susceptible to the effects of certain drugs than men and may need reduced dosages. Special care must also be taken during pregnancy as most drugs have an effect on the developing fetus, especially during the first trimester.

THE ROUTE OF ADMINISTRATION

In general, the more directly the drug is administered into the system, the smaller the dosage required to produce the effect. The least effective way of administering a drug is via the stomach, in the form of a pill, where a good portion of the drug may not be absorbed. Direct administration into the blood by IV is quicker and more direct than either intramuscular or subcutaneous injection, but is also potentially more dangerous and suitable to only certain types of medication.

The problems of faulty or incomplete absorption in the stomach are circumvented in certain compounds by sublingual (under-the-tongue) preparations where the rich blood supply of the vessels of the mouth is a rapid course of entry into the system.

The time at which a drug is taken also plays a major role in absorption. The stomach and GI tract absorb drugs more rapidly when they are free of food; consequently, a dose that is effective when taken on an empty stomach may be insufficiently absorbed and thus not entirely effective when the stomach is full. Unfortunately, many drugs are gastrointestinal irritants. This is especially true of aspirin and other pain-relieving and anti-inflammatory drugs. These drugs are better tolerated when taken with food or, if available, in a buffered combination.

TOLERANCE—THE LOSS OF DRUG EFFECT

Do drugs stop working after a time? One of the most common problems in using pain relievers is that the drugs do lose their effectiveness, often after only a short period of use. Tolerance is perhaps the most serious problem in the prescribing and use of narcotic pain relievers.

While the mechanisms involved in the development of tolerance are poorly understood, there is no question that it does occur, and especially in pain-relieving and tranquilizing drugs. In addition, tolerance is always associated with *cross-tolerance*, the loss of effect of pharmacologically similar drugs, particularly drugs that act at the same cell location. So if one type of narcotic pain-killer stops working, you can't just pick up and start with another: the effectiveness of all narcotics is diminished. Frequently the only recourse is to increase the dosage of a medication, a practice that can ultimately end in dependency or abuse.

DRUG BUILDUP AND DRUG DEPLETION

Drug toxicity—the effect of having too much active drug circulating in the system—can be caused in several different ways. One obvious manner is ingesting too much medication in too brief an interval. Another common próblem, especially in elderly and debilitated patients, is dysfunction of the organs responsible for the inactivation or excretion of the active drugs. (The term "active drug" refers to the particular molecular configuration of a drug where it is pharmacologically effective. The body, through various biochemical and physiological processes, can "inactivate" a drug. This work is generally done by enzyme systems in the liver.) In addition, any major disease, or the use of certain "competitive drugs" (they compete for enzyme systems in the liver), can prolong the body's normal breakdown of a drug and create toxicity.

On the other hand, there are certain drugs that prime or speed up metabolic breakdown processes. One way this is done is by stimulating the liver enzyme systems to inactivate drugs, thus preventing the attainment of effective blood levels for the therapeutic drugs. Basically, a drug cannot be effective unless an adequate blood level or "maintenance dose" is attained. Careful attention to the interval between the drug dosages, awareness of individual differences in metabolism, and scrupulous attention to the perceived "drug effect" will forestall many problems.

THE PLACEBO EFFECT

The term placebo comes directly from the Latin word meaning "I will please." The standard definition is "a medicine that has no drug effect; one that is given to humor the patient, tried for its psychological effect."

During the course of our medical training, we treated placebos with some contempt, as nonmedicine. Their use was confined to the occasional complaining patient whose pain or discomfort exceeded the expected allotment of complaints consistent with his or her medical problem.

Placebos are rarely given a fair shake in medicine, especially in recent years with the discovery of all sorts of wonder drugs. Why bother with a drug that does not really work? Are we to fool the patient into feeling better when we have drugs that are genuinely effective? It is wrong to think that the placebo is simply a means of deception. Under certain circumstances, placebos have alleviated pain, healed ulcers, corrected abnormalities, relieved hay fever, stopped coughs, and lowered blood pressure. It is pretty amazing that a pill with nothing in it can do all of this and more.

The placebo is not only a pill or substance for ingestion, insertion, or injection. The placebo effect dramatically illustrates the importance of the entire process of drug prescription, presentation, explanation, and, of course, patient expectation. The attitude of the doctor prescribing the medication and the care and emphasis given to the explanation of the medication play a most significant role in the ultimate efficacy of that medication. Many factors figure into the placebo effect, not the least of which are the patient's belief in the value of the medication and his willingness to take the medication in accordance with the prescribed regimen. The process of taking a medicine can be just as important as the medication itself.

There are biochemical aspects to the placebo effect of which we are just becoming aware. Besides the psychological elements of expectation, attitude, anticipation, and the need to please, there are some data to support the notion that the placebo effect may be enhanced by the endorphins. Naloxone,* a potent antagonist of morphine (it completely negates the effects of morphine), also negates the placebo effect. That is, if one is given morphine and a dose of Naloxone, the pain-reducing effects of morphine are blocked. It has been shown by some investigators that if one is given a placebo and told that it is morphine, a dose of Naloxone given after this "sugar pill" stops the placebo effect. This implies that there is some substance in the body that acts like morphine and may be responsible in part for the placebo effect. This substance may be endorphin, and thus endorphins probably play at least some role in the ancient placebo effect.

In summary, using medication intelligently requires an understanding of many factors and a desire to get the most value out of a particular drug. Swallowing a pill four times a day and expecting pain relief rarely works. A basic knowledge of drugs, their potential for abuse, and their benefits will serve to make you a better consumer of health care. Think before you swallow.

Chapter 14

PAIN AND NUTRITION: CONTROLLING
YOUR DIET

OBESITY: A NATIONAL EPIDEMIC

The very highly regarded cardiologist Paul Dudley White commented, "We were meant to be field animals. To race with the sun. To be in the open air. To be physically vigorous, and to eat only when hunger dictates." Dr. White was well aware of the special "nutritional disease" which plagues Americans. Unlike people in the underdeveloped nations, Americans do not suffer from vitamin deficiency or severe malnutrition—at least not when it is a measure of the amount of food we eat. The nutritional disease of America is obesity. The statistics are staggering. Fully 65 percent of all women between 50 and 60 and men between 38 and 48 are obese (at least ten pounds above their ideal body weight). As John Galbraith pointed out in *The Affluent Society,* "More die in the United States of too much food than too little."

Obesity contributes more to the chronicity of pain than many people realize. Every pound of excessive body weight is an additional load to be propelled through the tasks and activities of day-to-day living. This requires energy: physical, biochemical, and psychological—and energy is a very limited resource, especially if you are chronically in pain. The more weight, the greater the energy necessary to get you and your body through the day.

The mechanics of obesity add considerably to the perpetuation of pain. An excess of belly hung over one's belt is actually supported by the paraspinal muscles, a column of muscles running alongside the spine that helps maintain the postural integrity of the vertebral column. This extra burden of weight, carried about from dawn to dusk, places an additional pressure on the intervertebral disks. In a way, excess weight acts as a reverse form of traction, or antitraction. Instead of pulling the spine apart, providing more space for nerves to enter and exit, a large abdomen pushes the spine together, making it more difficult for nerves to enter and exit without being pressured or obstructed.

Additionally, obesity contributes to the psychological resistances that fuel the pain-go-round. Most people are fairly sensitive about their body image. Putting on weight, growing out of your clothes, and feeling less attractive than your "normal self" all distort the healthy mental image we all have of ourselves. It does not take long for a sense of helplessness to emerge accompanied by a reduction of energy and enthusiasm. You are left with less energy to push around more weight; every pound you gain helps fuel the pain-go-round.

Sitting at home, either bedridden or inactive, is a perfect setup for the development of an eating disorder. The prospect of eating (the prospect of pleasure) can become overwhelmingly powerful. Waiting around for the next meal is not a very dietetic way to spend the day.

Forty percent of all Americans are obese. Probably, a significantly higher proportion of chronic pain patients is overweight. Why is the incidence of this disorder so high? There are four major factors that contribute to the development of obesity. They are:

1. Genetic predisposition.
2. Overeating.
3. Inactivity.
4. The nature of the diet.

The pain sufferer is at increased risk to be significantly affected by all of these factors, with the exception of the first.

WHAT MAKES PEOPLE FAT?

"Imprisoned in every fat man a thin one is wildly signaling to be let out."   CYRIL CONNOLLY

Despite the theatrical ring of this statement, the cool reality is that it is not true. There are fat people who are fat, will remain fat, and may, if they choose, have children who will grow into fat adults. The propensity toward obesity does have genetic determinants. Not that your "weight fate" is cut and dried, stamped out in the chromosomes. Developmental factors do play a role. Yet studies of identical twins raised together or apart have demonstrated that identical twins with a predisposition to become obese will become obese despite differences in the environment in which they are raised. What this proves is that the apple may not fall far from the tree—unless, of course, it is rolling downhill. But don't lose all hope. While a propensity toward obesity does have *some* genetic determinants, there are many things that can be done to prevent the onset of calamity. The biologic tendency toward obesity is a significant but not necessarily a regulatory factor in the development of obesity.

EATING LESS? AND MORE . . .

Getting the pain patient to lose weight is extremely difficult. Many feel they eat minimally and "don't know where to cut back." Others feel that they cannot resist the constant temptation of food when they are sitting around all day. Still others complain of the lack of exercise: "I know I am in terrible shape, but when my pain gets better I will be able to exercise some more." The problem is, the pain does not get better, they just get fatter and subsequently more out of shape.

Many obese people feel helpless to control their weight. They do not think they overeat. Many probably do not. After a while they begin to wonder: is it possible to get fat simply by looking at food? Do fat people get more hungry than thin people when they think about or see food? According to Yale psychologist Judith Rodin, simply looking at food can produce biochemical and physiological changes that can result in increased food consumption. Dr. Rodin's research work has delineated the body's anticipatory response to external "food cues." Volunteer subjects were seated in front of a rack of sizzling steaks. Watching the steaks cook produced a secretion of insulin, which stimulated hunger. Dr. Rodin found that the "insulin response" was not uniform. Some people, notably obese individuals, showed a more pronounced "anticipatory food response" than others. Fat people physically and biochemically overreact to the thought of food.

Fat people stay fat because it is so easy to be coaxed, cajoled, or enticed into eating excessively. External food cues are everywhere and set off powerful internal processes that stimulate appetite. The more you eat, the fatter you get, and the more likely you are to continue overeating. Once the cycle is established, it is hard to turn it off.

What happens is that the visual image of food initiates an elaborate series of neurologic and endocrine events that ultimately terminate in a state of physical hunger. The brain, through its chemical messenger system, sends "dinner invitations" to tissues and organs throughout the body. Hunger is not simply an idea: it is a physical state of being.

If thinking about food stimulates hunger, then the idea of spending three weeks at home resting an aching back certainly provides ample opportunity to contemplate and eat. The more time you have to think about food, the more likely you are to stimulate your appetite. The danger of obesity lurks precariously in the shadows of rest and inactivity.

Pain and the Tendency to Overeat

Feelings of anxiety, tension, and boredom (all components of the pain cycle) are commonly associated with the tendency to develop an eating problem. Certain eating patterns may predominate. For the purpose of discussion, overeaters are divided into three major categories: munchers, stuffers, and speed freaks.

1. *Munchers* are free spirits. They avoid the restrictiveness of three squares and simply munch a bunch (of whatever) whenever they feel the urge.

People with pain problems are particularly susceptible to developing the munchies. The loss of structure in daily activities, the availability of food, and the general lack of vigorous activity that accompanies pain predisposes to hitting the refrigerator on a fairly regular basis.

The rationales for munching are as numerous as they are meager in substance. Many people claim they are not hungry: they eat because the food is available. Not "hungry enough" to eat a large meal, they simply nibble whenever they feel the urge, or simply whenever.

There are others who eat because they are "nervous" or "tense." Certainly, snacking provides something to do to help pass the time. It's terrific during commercials. It's also a great reason to go downstairs and see what's happening in the kitchen. Nonetheless, there are numerous substantial reasons why people with pain should avoid incessant eating:

1. In treating chronic pain the emphasis is on creating structure in the daily schedule. A predictable meal schedule is extremely useful.
2. Eating regular, planned meals is a considerably more reliable way to regulate the type and amount of food you eat. Unplanned snacks tend to be highly caloric and thus fattening.
3. High caloric snacking, especially of unrefined carbohydrates, causes the production of insulin, resulting in a stimulation of the appetite. The more sweets or treats you eat, the hungrier you become.
4. If you happen to have a weight problem, it is insidiously depressing to always have something in your mouth.

2. *Stuffers*. Bingeing, or eating too much at one sitting, is a particularly common form of overeating. The scenario usually involves individuals who, prior to the development of a pain problem, had little problem with their weight. Being more inactive over a period of months, they put on some weight. Generally not a lot, but enough to be annoying. To remedy the situation they decide to "diet." Rather than appropriately restricting the quantity of food at each meal, they elect to eliminate breakfast and lunch and focus solely on dinner. By the time the dinner rolls around, the faster is ravenous and may eat two to three times the normal allotment. After all, he isn't certain when his next meal is coming.

The disadvantages to this eating pattern are:

1. Taking all your calories in one meal overwhelms the body's capacity to handle the nutritional load. There is a greater likelihood that the food will be stored as fat.
2. Eating a single large meal is associated with increased serum cholesterol levels and decreased glucose tolerance.
3. It has been scientifically shown that weight can be maintained with 20 percent more calories if the calories are distributed throughout the day, rather than ingested in a single meal.
4. Anyone who watches you eat, when you do eat, will think that your obesity is a direct function of the amount you eat. Embarrassed about having people watch you, there is a tendency to go underground, eat when no one is looking. We call this the closet gourmet syndrome.

Table 1
Suggested weights for men by height and body frame

Height In. (cm)	Small frame lbs. (kg)	Average frame lbs. (kg)	Large frame lbs. (kg)
60 (152)	106 (48)	117 (53)	130 (59)
61 (155)	110 (50)	121 (55)	133 (60)
62 (157)	114 (52)	125 (57)	137 (62)
63 (160)	118 (54)	129 (59)	141 (64)
64 (163)	122 (55)	133 (60)	145 (66)
65 (165)	126 (57)	137 (62)	149 (68)
66 (168)	130 (59)	142 (64)	155 (70)
67 (170)	134 (61)	147 (67)	161 (73)
68 (173)	139 (63)	151 (69)	166 (75)
69 (175)	143 (65)	155 (70)	170 (77)
70 (178)	147 (67)	159 (72)	174 (79)
71 (180)	150 (68)	163 (74)	178 (81)
72 (183)	154 (70)	167 (76)	183 (83)
73 (185)	158 (72)	171 (78)	188 (85)
74 (188)	162 (74)	175 (79)	192 (87)
75 (191)	165 (75)	178 (81)	195 (89)
76 (193)	168 (76)	181 (82)	198 (90)
77 (196)	172 (78)	185 (84)	202 (92)
78 (198)	175 (79)	188 (85)	205 (93)

3. *Speed Freak*. Fat people have a tendency to eat too fast. People with pain are uncomfortable sitting in one place too long. The combination is trouble. Slowing down your delivery, making mealtime last longer, can actually take pounds off. Besides, it's nice to taste what you put in your mouth.

INACTIVITY

Controlling your weight involves a whole lot more than just watching what you eat. There is a very slim chance, about 5 percent, of losing weight solely on the basis of dietary restrictions without exercise and behavior modification. Inactivity, the consequence of a sedentary life, greatly reduces the normal caloric requirement of our bodies and is thus a major factor in the development of obesity.

Table 2
Suggested weights for women by height and body frame

Height In. (cm)	Small frame lbs. (kg)	Average frame lbs. (kg)	Large frame lbs. (kg)
58 (147)	94 (43)	102 (46)	110 (50)
59 (150)	97 (44)	105 (48)	114 (52)
60 (152)	100 (45)	109 (49)	118 (54)
61 (155)	104 (47)	112 (51)	121 (55)
62 (157)	107 (49)	115 (52)	125 (57)
63 (160)	110 (50)	118 (54)	128 (58)
64 (163)	113 (51)	122 (55)	132 (60)
65 (165)	116 (53)	125 (57)	135 (61)
66 (168)	120 (54)	129 (59)	139 (63)
67 (170)	123 (56)	132 (60)	142 (64)
68 (173)	126 (57)	136 (62)	146 (66)
69 (175)	130 (59)	140 (64)	151 (69)
70 (178)	133 (60)	144 (65)	156 (71)
71 (180)	137 (62)	148 (67)	161 (73)
72 (183)	141 (64)	152 (69)	166 (75)
73 (185)	145 (66)	156 (71)	171 (78)
74 (188)	149 (68)	160 (73)	176 (80)
75 (191)	153 (69)	164 (74)	181 (82)

Since 1958, the National Research Council has actually lowered the recommended daily caloric allowances for normal adults by approximately 10 percent. The reason is that people expend less energy during the course of a day, perhaps an adverse consequence (at least in terms of weight control) of the numerous labor-saving devices that have proliferated in our society.

HOW MANY CALORIES ARE ENOUGH?

There are many tables available to document the number of calories a person should eat in the course of a day. Some tables take into account height, weight, and age, and recommend a daily allowance (see Tables 1 and 2). But measuring calories without taking into account "output," or how the calories are spent, does not provide an accurate measure of metabolic balance. Whatever comes in has to be measured in terms of what gets used. If you eat it and don't "burn it," then you wear it until you do.

For example, let's examine Table 3.*

Table 3
How much is enough?

Your ideal body weight $\times$ (10) light activity $\Big\}$ ideal calories
                     (15) moderate activity $=$ to maintain
                     (20) heavy activity   body weight

If you are between the ages of

25 and 34	subtract zero
35 and 44	subtract 100
44 and 54	subtract 200
54 and 64	subtract 300
65+	subtract 400

The above table is designed to determine the number of calories needed to maintain an individual "ideal" body weight. For example, an obese fifty-year-old woman who should weigh 120 pounds (but does weigh 160 pounds) would maintain her ideal weight, 120 pounds, by keeping moderately active and eating:

$120 \times (15) = 1800$ calories
less 200 calories for age $= 1600$ calories, her ideal daily allowance.

If her activity schedule went from moderate to light, then her caloric requirement would fall 600 calories, or 36 percent!
$120 \times (10) = 1200$ calories less 200 calories for age $= 1000$ calories.

CASE EXAMPLE

Mrs. Goldberg is a healthy, active, forty-five-year-old woman. She has three children, ages twenty, seventeen, and nine. She lives in a four-bedroom home, which she keeps up. She works part time as a receptionist in a doctor's office, plays tennis twice a week, and is

* Adapted from *Nutrition and Obesity*, by Richard Atkinson, M.D., from "The Medicine Called Nutrition," a CDC International Monograph (1979).

generally on the go fourteen hours a day. Mrs. Goldberg is comfortable with her weight, is not obese. The following daily menu is fairly typical:

MRS. GOLDBERG'S MENU

BREAKFAST	CALORIES
Coffee and sugar	30
1 slice bread with 1 pat butter and 1 teaspoon jam	106
4 large prunes	172
	308

LUNCH	
Bacon, lettuce, tomato sandwich	282
8 ounces lemonade	105
Coconut custard pie (⅙ of 9-inch pie)	355
	742

COCKTAIL	
3½ ounces muscatel, port	160

DINNER	
Chicken noodle soup	62
Hot roast beef, with gravy	430
4 medium mushrooms, fried	78
Baked potato with butter	200
Cauliflower with mayonnaise sauce	110
Hard roll with butter	145
	1025

SNACK	
20 peanuts	160
1 medium apple	87
	247	TOTAL 2482

Since she is heavily active, her calculated daily requirements are:

$140 \times (20) = 2800$ calories
less 200 for age $= 2600$ calories

So her regular diet leaves ample room for occasional extra snacks without the danger of weight gain. Her caloric intake and active lifestyle are well balanced.

In the course of events, Mrs. Goldberg slips while getting out of the car and sprains her back. She goes to bed for three weeks with virtually no activity. Her estimated caloric requirement (see Table 3), based on light activity:

$$140 \times (10) = 1400, \text{ less } 200 \text{ for age} = 1200$$
estimated daily intake   2400 (same diet)
excess of intake over output   1200 calories

It will not take long for Mrs. Goldberg to gain weight. If you examine her diet, there isn't much margin for caloric reduction. We believe it is unreasonable to assume that the average person, especially one who is afflicted by a significant pain problem, will be able to strip all unnecessary carbohydrates and fats from her diet. An occasional piece of pie, a couple of cookies, or a breakfast roll are too highly valued as treats to totally eliminate from a regular diet. We all anticipate and welcome a food reward from time to time.

The solution to weight gain requires a multidimensional approach, one that includes a restructuring of the diet as well as an increase in physical activity. The first step in entering into an exercise program is to clarify your activity restrictions with your personal physician. Find out exactly what you are able to do to increase the expenditure of energy so that you can comfortably balance "excessive" calories.

It is estimated that walking briskly (three to four miles per hour) expends 5.2 calories a minute. While it is not necessary for everyone to walk that fast, the table below provides a basis for understanding the exercise equivalent of calories, and how the burning of calories results in weight loss.

Begin to consider long-term changes in your activity level by including regular exercise such as walking, swimming, or jogging in your schedule. Increasing the amount of exercise you get can do more to "cure" obesity than all the fad diets in town.

TIPS ON DIETS FOR THE VERY SEDENTARY

"If you have found the habit of checking on every new diet that comes along, you will find that, mercifully, they all blur together, leaving you with only one definite piece of information: french fried potatoes are out."
                                                                JEAN KERR

Table 4
Days required to lose 5 to 25 pounds
by walking* and lowering daily calorie intake†

Minutes of + walking	Reduction of calories per day (in kcal)	Days to lose 5 lbs.	Days to lose 10 lbs.	Days to lose 15 lbs.	Days to lose 20 lbs.	Days to lose 25 lbs.
30	400	27	54	81	108	135
30	600	20	40	60	80	100
30	800	16	32	48	64	80
30	1,000	13	26	39	52	65
45	400	23	46	69	92	115
45	600	18	36	54	72	90
45	800	14	28	42	56	70
45	1,000	12	24	36	48	60
60	400	21	42	63	84	105
60	600	16	32	48	64	80
60	800	13	26	39	52	65
60	1,000	11	22	33	44	55

Tip 1: You can't fool Mother Nature: she keeps everything in balance. Most American diets are too high in fats (40 to 50 percent of the daily calories, while experts recommend 33 percent, especially for the sedentary). Avoid fat-rich pastries and desserts, foods made with egg yolks, and whole milk, cream, and cheese. High-fat foods are high in calories, cholesterol, and low-density lipids (fats that are thought to play a role in the development of heart disease).

Tip 2: Even if you're not moving, try to keep your bowels moving: eat fiber.

Hippocrates, the father of medicine, recommended unbolted wheat meal bread for its salutary effects on the bowels. Fiber is present in bran, grains, fruits, and vegetables; it is an important element of a balanced diet because, among other things, it adds bulk to the intestinal contents. Fiber absorbs water, increasing the mass of the stool and accelerating the movement of food through the bowel.

* Walking briskly (3.5–4.0 mph), calculated at 5.2 cal/minute.
† *Exercise Equivalents of Foods,* by Frank Konishi, Southern Illinois University Press, Carbondale and Edwardsville, Feffer & Simons, Inc., London and Amsterdam, 1973.

While there is no evidence that high-fiber diets aid in weight reduction, there is no question that a high-fiber diet requires more chewing and tends to satisfy hunger quicker.

Tip 3: When you are spending time sitting around it always seems like a good time to eat. By planning your snacks to include natural, unprocessed foods such as fruits and vegetables, you can avoid the temptation of indulging in more caloric snacks.

Tip 4: Do not eat all your calories at one sitting, or you will overload your body's capacity to handle calories effectively. As a result, more calories get stored as fat. You will do better eating at regular times.

Tip 5: Drink coffee and alcohol only in moderation. Coffee contains high amounts of caffeine which, in excess, can increase anxiety and restlessness.

Alcohol is a potent drug which can be easily abused, especially in situations of extreme stress and pressure. It is not unusual to see an exacerbation of a quiescent alcohol problem in a person who develops a chronic pain syndrome. The pressure of living in pain can stir up some dull roots.

In addition, alcohol is highly caloric. A four-ounce glass of wine has eighty-five calories, a one-and-a-half-ounce shot of whiskey 125 calories, and a can of beer 175 calories. Restricting your diet means decreasing your alcohol consumption.

Tip 6: Since you may have to start eating less, pay more attention to what you do eat. Find menus that use low-calorie ingredients, and try including herbs and spices as flavoring instead of adding salt. Avoid the sauces and condiments that are overly rich. Learn to steam vegetables; they'll taste so much better you won't need sauces. Try using lemon juice to perk up flavors. Use safflower oil (high in polyunsaturated fats) in your cooking. Experiment!

Chapter 15

THE ART OF RELAXATION

STRESS AND THE TENSION HEADACHE

In general, people have come to take the tension headache for granted. Listen to enough advertisements and you come to believe that two aspirin tablets are a natural chaser to either a hard day at the office or a houseful of screaming kids. Just living, putting up with the minor annoyances of life, should be reason enough to get a hummer of a headache.

Wrong. Despite the media blitz, headaches are *not* a normal physiological response to a hard day. Headaches are abnormal; they are symptoms that reflect changes in the mind and body.

The classic tension headache, or "crown of thorns," is one of the most common pain responses to excessive stress. Muscles of the neck and shoulder girdle, under the force of prolonged contraction, tense up, and go into spasm. The pain rapidly spreads up the back of the head, darts around the ears, and ends up throbbing right between your eyes. It is the kind of headache that persists throughout the day, generally getting worse in the late afternoon. The typical tension headache gradually improves as one relaxes in the evening (partially leaving the stress and strain of the day behind). By relieving the undercurrent of mental pressure that pulsates throughout the course of a hectic day, the muscles you unconsciously spent the afternoon tying into knots (especially in the neck, shoulder girdle, and lower back) begin to loosen up.

Surprisingly, the stress tension cycle does not cut off when you retire. In our experience, patients with persistent tension headache often experience the greatest distress in the early morning. Additionally, they don't sleep well (if at all) and wake up dull, fatigued, and more haggard than when they retired. If relaxation eases tension, then why shouldn't sleep break the cycle?

Sleep is not necessarily relaxing; it can be outright exhausting. The stress and tension of daily living do not disappear when you close your eyes. For many, the absence of conscious distraction enhances the focus on conflict and problems. The mental mechanisms do not turn off (as much as we would like them to) but replay the day's or week's or even year's most trying, perplexing, or otherwise troublesome memories.

Troubled people, especially those with persistent pain, have troubled sleep. The agony of the day does not go away by simply closing your eyes.

BUILDING UP BODY TENSION

Body tension begins as mental tension. In the stressful environment of our electronically hyperactive world, the pace of life can easily accelerate beyond an individual's coping capacity. Minor life events, such as being late, fighting with your spouse, offending a client, being in pain, or even the anticipation of pain, can create mental tension. As tension accumulates, an unconscious transformation from mental to physical energy occurs. You may begin to grind your teeth, clench your fists, tense up muscles of the neck and shoulder girdle.

Suddenly the pain appears. Rather dramatically, you begin to feel bad. Muscles stimulated into chronic states of contraction go into spasm. Spasm is painful. As muscles contract, they release compounds that intensify the pain. Pain intensifies and creates more tension and spasm. A cycle is established. If the muscle (or any part of the anatomy) has been previously damaged as a result of injury or disease (specifically arthritis or the degenerative diseases of aging), then the resulting pain may be extraordinarily severe and the cycle unremitting.

Muscular contraction is only one response to excessive stress. There are many. The human alerting response was first described by Walter Cannon, who coined the term "flight or fight" response and emphasized the adaptive importance of the biological process. By quickly and automatically preparing to either fight or run, the human is able to make appropriate responses to danger in the environment. Just the mental perception (or imagination) of danger causes an outpouring of hormones and compounds that speeds up our physiological process. For example, the awareness of danger (in whatever concrete or abstract form) stimulates an "adrenergic," or alerting response. The nature of the danger is irrelevant; we can be stressed as much by the sight of a furious bear as by the unpleasant memory of an angry encounter. Whatever the source of stress, the biological response is remarkably similar: our system is primed for action.

The Stress Response

The brain communicates the stress response through the autonomic (involuntary) nervous system that controls the automatic activities, such as circulation of blood, breathing, digestion of food, and excretion of wastes. By overstimulating the involuntary nervous system, living under conditions of ever-present stress, we produce changes in the functions of our body. Increased heart rate, high blood pressure, excessive sweating, poor digestion, and respiratory problems are all produced by excessive stress. The end result is the development of disease. While the exact mechanisms have not been elaborated, scientists feel certain that stress contributes to the development of many major diseases.

Chronic pain is a common manifestation of stress-created disease. As the stress-tension cycle accelerates, it can intensify the pain of stomach distress, ulcer disease, angina (heart pain), or chronic arthritis. Stress, as we stated earlier, is the constant companion of chronic pain. Living in pain is a stress of the highest order, but it is not the only source of stress. For many, just living in our modern world is emotionally draining. In a way, our biological equipment— the autonomic nervous system—is too sensitive. With all the danger around us, the inherent conflict of living, it's a bit ironic that the archaic biological mechanism designed to protect us from danger should become a major health problem.

Pain and the Conditioned Response

Many years ago, Dr. B. F. Skinner of Harvard University demonstrated through a series of animal experiments that behavior could be controlled by changes in the environment. Skinner worked with pigeons. He rewarded them with food for pecking at a certain key on a keyboard. The animal would expect a food reward for the appropriate behavior. When confronted with the keyboard the animal would peck at the key, begin to salivate, and await his reward. Eventually, Skinner removed the food reward, but that didn't change the bird's behavior; he continued to peck away expecting the food reward: his behavior had become conditioned. This shaping of voluntary behavior is called operant conditioning.

For many people with chronic pain the expectation of pain produces a conditioned response (pain behavior) which over time is experienced as pain. As humans, we become conditioned to expect pain and can actually experience pain as a function of our expectation. Even in cases where there is a peripheral source of pain (an acute injury or sprain, for example), the anticipation of pain intensifies the experience. We have the capacity to accelerate or reduce the pain experience as a function of a conditioned response.

The conditioned response is not limited to voluntary behavior but also effects the involuntary nervous system. Dr. Neil Miller of the Rockefeller Institute applied theories of operant conditioning to studies of the autonomic nervous system. His research pioneered the clinical use of biofeedback training. Mental techniques that altered heart rate, reduced muscle contraction and spasm, lowered skin temperature, even lowered blood pressure, were developed. The use of biofeedback apparatus allowed the individual to mechanically monitor the changes he could mentally induce in his bodily functions. The anticipatory and regulatory powers of the mind could be scientifically verified and electronically documented. The wonders of the human mind, the ability of the brain to influence the function of the body, could at last be verified. And so we know that the mind holds the power to decondition the conditioned response and break the cycle of tension and pain.

THE NEED FOR RELAXATION

Stress, tension, and pain are the three horsemen of the modern Apocalypse; drugs and alcohol (substance abuse) are the fourth. Breaking the cycle of stress, tension, and pain requires an effort at self-enforced relaxation. Simply taking vacations will not help, especially if they are filled with hectic scurrying about or backbreaking schedules. Time away from the strain of daily living cannot be deferred until two weeks in August. The occasion to depart from the daily strains must occur on a regular and predictable basis. Minivacations, little periods of relief, should be included in the day-to-day scheduling of your life.

Integrating relaxation into your daily schedule will protect against excessive stress. People who can relax function more effectively, stay healthier, and ultimately, all other things being equal, live longer.

Successful people, those who have made substantial professional achievement, are frequently found to enjoy the best health and be most comfortable with their personal and emotional life. Some documentation of the "healthy executive syndrome" has been provided by a study from a major insurance company, which found that top-level executives of the nation's largest companies had less stress-related illness (angina, high blood pressure, arthritis, chronic pain) than a comparable group of men matched for age and weight (men who had less responsible jobs and presumably less stressful lives). The higher-level executives were generally healthier and more fit, complained less about excessive stress, and appeared to enjoy their demanding jobs. Many admitted to using relaxation techniques to manage stress. For the busy executive, stress control was not a convenience but a matter of necessity and survival. Virtually all of these chief executives had jobs that required working ten to fourteen hours a day. They had developed techniques to reduce the tedium and tension of their daily responsibilities. Excessive stress was rarely a problem; they enjoyed their jobs, found work exciting and vigorous, and could perform competently and tirelessly for extended periods.

In our experience active people who can actively control their lives are most healthy. As pain debilitates, it cripples the power to cope with the pressure and stress of life. The chronically ill person who is conditioned to live in pain has conditioned himself to dwell in a state of excessive stress. Permanent changes cannot occur unless the stress-tension cycle can be intercepted.

What Is Relaxation?

Many people mistake fatigue, exhaustion, or even depression for relaxation. Patients will often report feeling "relaxed" when in fact they are in a state of intense muscular contraction or under severe mental stress. These people are not pretending or lying; they do not know how to relax.

Just lying down, resting, or sitting still will not produce a state of relaxation. Nor will telling someone to "take it easy," "relax," or "hang loose" produce any change in his or her physical or emotional status. Relaxation is a self-induced process of progressive mental and physical conditioning that results in a "new" and dramatically tempered mental and physical state.

Relaxation techniques—the various methods for controlling the involuntary nervous system—are not unique to twentieth century technology. Centuries ago, long before biofeedback and the newer techniques of relaxation treatment, dramatic claims for controlling bodily function came from the eastern cultures, especially the meditative techniques of yoga and Zen Buddhism. The Indians, who practiced yoga for centuries in an effort to achieve the greatest possible control of mind over body, have used the power of concentration for lowering body temperature to actually slow the heartbeat. Scientific studies conducted with Zen monks have demonstrated actual physiological changes including decreased oxygen consumption, lower blood pressure, and lower metabolism.

Dr. Herbert Benson, director of the Hypertension Division of the Beth Israel Hospital in Boston, studied a group of people competent in the practice of Transcendental Meditation, a modern derivative of the ancient meditative state. He set up experiments to document the effects of meditation and found practitioners of the art could decrease their rate of metabolism and attain a state of altered consciousness. Uniformly, their oxygen consumption decreased, alpha, or slow, brain waves increased (a sign of mental relaxation), and blood lactate (a compound alleged to produce attacks of anxiety when injected into human subjects) decreased. Additionally, all the practitioners of the meditative art, many of whom had been doing it for ten or fifteen years, had low blood pressure. Dr. Benson concluded "that lowered oxygen consumption, heart rate, respiration and blood lactate are indicative of decreased activity of the sympathetic nervous system and represent a hypometabolic, or restful state. What is inferred is that these physiologic changes are reproducible through the techniques of any number of popularized meditative techniques and that the responses are antagonistic to the harmful effects of excessive stress."

PUTTING THEORY TO PRACTICE

There is no permanent, absolute, unchangeable truth; what we should pursue is the most convenient arrangement of our ideas. The same can be said for relaxation therapies. No matter how good or innovative, for them to prove worthwhile we must be able to use their techniques to our advantage. The simpler an idea, the more closely it resembles the routine activities of daily life, the more likely one is to incorporate that idea into the course of daily activity. The easier something is to do, the more likely one is to do it.

Where meditation and relaxation techniques are applied to the treatment of anxiety, pain, and other physical and emotional illness, there is a high risk of failure. It seems that few, if any, individuals can benefit from these techniques. The reasons are:

1. People do not adequately learn and master the techniques of relaxation. They are subtle and difficult, and attention to detail and long periods of concentrated effort are essential to their mastery. Few people have the time, energy, and effort to dedicate themselves to these self-healing techniques.
2. As enthusiasm in attempting the techniques wanes, so does one's effort to persist with difficult tasks. Many people quit long before getting the technique mastered. If something doesn't help, "why should I keep doing it?"
3. Even under the best conditions, improvement is not sudden or dramatic. Change, especially control of the stress response and the pain-tension cycle, occurs slowly, subtly, and only after a whole lot of effort.

Learning Deep Relaxation

Teaching a person with pain the art of relaxation is like telling someone who is sitting in the dentist's chair, hearing the drill buzzing, to relax. Fingers clenched tenaciously around the arms of the chair, thighs tense, the patient sits rigidly with a half-crazed daze staring anxiously into the overhead light; and the doctor matter-of-factly says, "Relax! You're too tense." When it comes to pain we're all pretty bad actors. Learning to grin and bear it is fine, provided that it's not your teeth that are being drilled.

Nonetheless, the dentist or whoever else advises you to relax when confronted with the prospect of pain knows something quite valuable. Genuine relaxation can actually lower the experience of pain. Being able to change the states of one's consciousness to slow down the alerting, or sympathetic, response can break the pain-tension cycle. Unfortunately, talking about it is a lot easier than doing it.

Special techniques must be implemented to achieve relaxation. We recommend a combination of meditation and muscle relaxation which we call deep relaxation. It is based upon the successive enhancement of three critical factors:

1. attaining and then maintaining a state of physical comfort,
2. achieving mental calm and deep physical relaxation, and
3. diffusion of the pain.

Mastering each of the steps is essential to learning the art of relaxation. Implementing each step in succession is critical. While there are many techniques for achieving relaxation, all methods require patience, persistence, and constant practice—the three p's of successful relaxation training.

THE SETTING

While an accomplished yogi can sit self-absorbed in the midst of the congested Casbah and attain unity with his inner self, the ordinary person requires a greater degree of isolation and tranquillity to get started. Do not underestimate the power of distraction, especially as it applies to pain. Any stimulus in the environment can interrupt the initiation of deep relaxation. Select a quiet spot. It doesn't necessarily have to be your bed or living room couch. A spot on the lawn (provided the temperature is appropriate), a carpeted floor, and my personal favorite, the rope hammock, are all excellent selections. Avoid sound, especially television and radio. Even soothing "beautiful music" is detrimental, as it causes external or environmental focusing. Choose your spot carefully to ensure maximum comfort and privacy.

ALLOW TIME

Time for deep relaxation should be scheduled into the day. It seems a bit ironic having to schedule relaxation, but many of us lack sufficient motivation and discipline to spontaneously initiate this focused activity.

One busy executive with chronic tension headache decided to take fifteen minutes at 2 P.M. every day to practice his technique. He knew that 2 P.M. was a critical time, for it marked the point where tension was beginning to be built up sufficiently to initiate the spasm in his neck and shoulder that inevitably led to his five-o'clock headache. So each day at 2 P.M., the executive would excuse himself from what he was doing, retreat to the quiet isolation of his office, recline in his oversized desk chair, and go through fifteen minutes of meditation. People in the office initially thought it strange to see the boss retreat into his office, shut the door, cut off all calls, and seclude himself every afternoon precisely at 2 P.M. But no one complained when his crotchety, arrogant demeanor—so long considered just a part of his personality—began to mellow. Best of all for the executive, his headaches all but disappeared—not suddenly or overnight, but over a period of six months he noticed significant improvement. Still, every day at 2 P.M., he persisted in his meditative practice. He believed meditation helped him and as long as he practiced, the headaches were well controlled.

It's hard to feel "in the mood" for deep relaxation, and it's all but impossible to achieve relaxation without plenty of regular practice. Be smart: schedule your relaxation time.

GETTING COMFORTABLE

Finding a position that you can remain in for a period of at least fifteen minutes is an important prerequisite to relaxation. Many pain patients have a hard time finding a comfortable spot. Everybody has his own technique for avoiding pain. For most people this means squirming around a lot. But restlessness is one sure obstacle to achieving deep relaxation. Fidgeting about, stretching your legs and arms, squirming from one place to another, all break the spell of relaxation.

The expert meditators can tuck their legs underneath their bottoms, sit perfectly still on a hard floor, and go to work. If you have a pain problem you may find this out of the question; lying calmly on the couch may be hard enough. Therefore you may need to make some special preparations prior to attempting deep relaxation.

If you have a low back problem, try placing a firm pillow under the small of your back. Move the pillow up and down until you hit a spot that provides comfortable support. Once the pillow is placed, leave it. Avoid fidgeting. Allow your back to "settle" around the pillow. For cervical neck problems, a pillow under the neck and head is excellent support. Massaging the painful area, stretching and gently kneading the muscles will help ease muscle tension and is good preparation for practicing relaxation.

Temporomandibular joint (the hinge that connects the upper and lower jaw together) pain presents a special challenge for loosening up the neck and jaw. Finding and maintaining a well-supported but soft reclining position for the head and neck is critical. A brief fingertip massage of the temporal region will help "loosen the jaw" and sensitize the joint to the relaxation process.

Special effort should be made to put the painful area at complete rest. Using a heating pad during the relaxation exercise is perfectly permissible. It may enhance the level of muscle relaxation. Anything that increases the level of personal comfort is fair game, provided that you can implement the effect yourself. Try to minimize your reliance on other people; relaxation is a private matter. Practice at your convenience and do not rely on others to help you.

The goal of getting comfortable is finding a position where you will be able to "sink" into the spot of your choice. Deep relaxation requires concomitant muscle relaxation. The ability to diffuse the pain is dependent upon the body's ability to imaginatively sink into the surface it's lying on. Your body should be able to attain a state of suspended animation. Quiet and comfort are essential to this process.

FOCUSING

Focusing is the critical mental process by which you choose an object to dwell on during the process of relaxation. Getting one's mind off chronic pain is absolutely essential. In the classic system of yoga, as described in the writings of Patañjali (who classified a series of traditional meditative practices in India), the critical element is concentration on a single point. This point could be a physical object or thought, a single mental image. Absorbing your mental energies in a single focus creates an aura of calm—a self-absorption of rest, tranquillity, and acceptance. The goal is to come to peace with yourself, ease your anxiety, calm your mind and body.

Controlling pain requires accepting the presence of pain. By not fighting against pain, simply allowing a painful sensation to peacefully exist within you, you can limit the potential debilitating struggle of fighting off a headache or overreacting to a morning backache.

We have created very simple exercises which, if practiced correctly, can help you create a new sense of relaxation.

EXERCISE 1

Getting Comfortable

1. Lie down in a comfortable, quiet spot.
2. Begin to breathe deeply. Gently fill your chest, allowing your chest cavity to expand. Feel your back widening and your shoulders rising. Hold the air for a count of three. Slowly release the air from your chest.
3. Continue breathing slowly and rhythmically.
4. Think of a pleasant scene, one free of pain and discomfort. Imagine yourself in an activity where you are totally enjoying yourself.
5. Spend a full *five* minutes lying down and gently breathing. Stick to the single mental image. Begin to imagine yourself sinking into the surface you're lying on.
6. Were you able to get your thoughts focused? If not, what problems or thoughts got in the way (distractions)?
   1.
   2.
   3.
7. Repeat the process of focusing three times today. Try to correct the *distractions*.

EXERCISE 2

Blowing Off the Pain Vapors

1. Find a comfortable spot to sit.
2. Stay perfectly still. Stop all movement.
3. Concentrate on your breathing. Imagine visualizing the air as it leaves your nostrils. Pretend the air leaving your nostrils is bright red, filled with the venom of your pain.

4. Breathe in, hold the breath for several seconds, then breathe out fully and deeply. Watch the "red" clouds drift away.
5. Concentrate only on your breathing as you lie motionless.

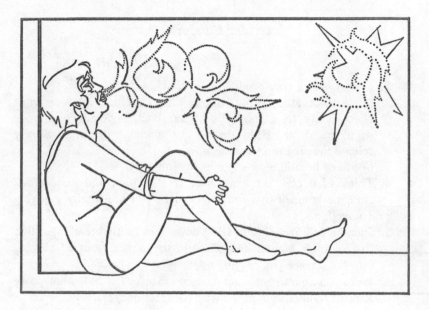

Blowing off the pain vapors.

EXERCISE 3

Focusing On The Ideal Image

1. Lie down in a comfortable, quiet spot.
2. Think of a calm and restful scene. Perhaps it's a beach, with the sound of the waves producing a rhythmic lulling. Or a peaceful hillside, or a secluded lake.
3. Fix the scene in your mind. Focus on the "feelings" of your image. Feel the surf or breeze, smell the fragrance of the scene. Involve all five senses. Mentally lose yourself in the sensations of the image.

4. Put yourself into the scene. Become part of the fantasy. Totally
   absorb yourself in the tranquillity.

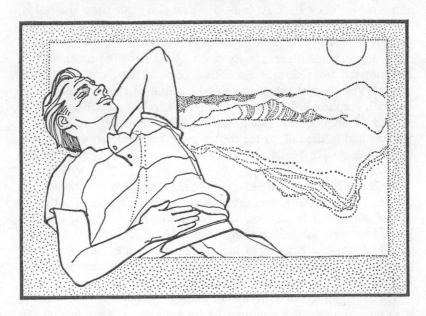

"Imaging."

Each of the three exercises should be practiced two or three times
a day. You can do all three in one sitting and repeat this three times
during the day, or you may find it easier to do them at different
times. Use your own judgment. Remember, this is a process for relaxation. Don't become so attentive to the detail of doing the exercises that you forget the goal—relaxation.

The exercises get progressively easier to do. Once mastered they
can be done very quickly and easily and should become a routine
part of your day.

A CASE HISTORY OF RELAXATION THERAPY: MEL AND THE
BIG ORANGE ONE

The man most responsible for the invention of color therapy is
Mel Ostrow. In the course of treatment, Mel told me the history of
his headache problem and, significantly, how he came to develop
color therapy.

As an allergic child he had been troubled by sinus headaches. According to Mel, his mother dragged him to every bigshot doctor along New York's Park Avenue. He saw allergists, nose specialists, internists, even a guy who specialized in infectious disease. For years he took a handful of pills three times a day. Some made him drowsy, some dopey, while others simply dried up his nose (so much so that Mel suffered from chronic nosebleed because his membranes were so dry). An allergist actually drained his sinuses (most unpleasant), but still, despite all the treatments, his headaches persisted. Nothing seemed to help. Every spring, as the roses bloomed, he began to wheeze, and in the fall, as the molds grew, he would sneeze. The allergies inflamed his sinuses, producing an almost constant frontal headache.

Mel's mother, herself an allergic woman, took his afflictions quite personally. As often is the case, she felt guilty. Mel had inherited her problems, her headaches. She was in anguish at the sight of his bloodshot eyes, the bulbous red nose, and his drowsy, half-opened eyelids. When she discovered his adolescent friends had nicknamed him "Dopey," she lost patience and vowed to finally resolve his allergies. Mel was to stop sneezing, whatever the cost.

She took him to see a prominent allergy specialist at Mount Sinai, who after thoroughly examining Mel assured Mrs. Ostrow that her son had an allergic sinusitis which was undoubtedly causing his headaches. Further, he predicted that Melvin would probably "outgrow" the allergies and cure himself.

The learned doctor had correctly assessed Melvin, but had grossly underestimated Mrs. Ostrow's guilt. She was adamant: Melvin had to stop sneezing. The allergies had gone far enough. If they didn't stop calling her son "Dopey," he might begin to believe it.

"Doctor," she exclaimed, "you simply have to do something. My son suffers terribly and you tell him he'll grow out of it. All night he's up sneezing, he's constantly blowing his nose, and oh, the headaches, what headaches he gets!"

"Your son gets headaches?" he inquired.

"Of course, he takes aspirin all day for the headaches."

At this point Mel spoke up. "Listen, Mom, the headaches aren't so bad. I can live with them."

"No. You're falling asleep in class from all the medication, and something has to be done."

The white-haired allergist peered over his glasses at this pathetic lad with the constantly dripping nose. "Well, I suppose we could irrigate and drain the sinuses."

Immediately Mrs. Ostrow rose, and a look of relief flashed across her face. "You see, there *is* something you can do. There is a treatment. Good, when can he start?"

For the next six months, Melvin had his sinuses irrigated and drained on a regular monthly basis. To say he hated the procedure of having tubes stuck up through his nose to lodge somewhere in the frontal sinus would be a gross understatement. It hurt far more than sneezing all the time, and he could never understand why he had to treat something that would heal by itself.

A curious transformation occurred in Mel's attitude. He began to look forward, to actually anticipate the sinus headaches. He found having the headaches far less traumatic than getting the cure. Getting the headaches was reassuring. They were familiar.

Whenever he felt a headache coming, he imagined a giant cloud engulfing his head and he would color the headache. Each one was different. Some were red and warm, others were pink and light and fluffy, while others were gray and ominous. When the headache began, Mel would sit back, relax, and get into the headache. He would try to understand the pain, feel it engulf him and cascade around him, and become part of the pain. The color gave the headache a personality. Mel felt it made the pain less impersonal and threatening. As a result the headaches were less intense, less persistent. For the most part, the pain would go largely unnoticed.

Unknown to him at the time, Mel had stumbled upon "color therapy," a type of relaxation training. He had effectively used a mental mechanism to control his response to the headache. As a result he was not panicked or frightened by the headache, but basically accepted the pain, raised his threshold through mental powers, and eventually overcame the pain.

The treatment is paradoxical in that it is based on pretending that something "bad" is in fact "good." Giving the headache color and imagery, imagining it as a cloud passing through the head, served to defuse it. Mel had learned to fool his head by seeing the pain as a friend and not an enemy. Eventually he outgrew his allergies, stopped his seasonal sneezing and wheezing, and after junior high school no one ever referred to him as "Dopey" again. But what did endure was Mel's color therapy.

Chapter 16

PAIN AND EXERCISE

THE PROCESS OF ACTIVE CONDITIONING

Fully 50 percent of chronic pain can be traced to muscle spasm and binding, according to Dr. Hans Kraus of New York. Sore, pinched muscles are painful to move and many people just do not move them. It is natural to allow sore muscles to rest. Inactivity feels better, but nothing can be worse than letting chronically painful muscles fall into disuse. As one can see by the following chart; a vicious cycle of pain, inactivity, and eventual atrophy will occur.

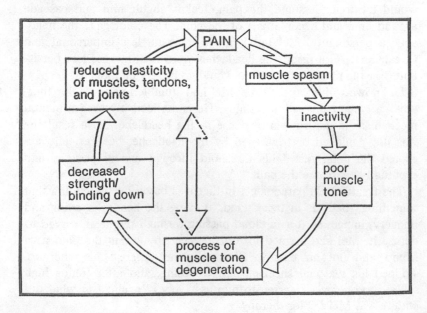

From pain to disability.

Attention to muscle health can play a part in reducing chronic pain. We can divide our concern about muscles into three areas:

1. *Posture*—the "positioning" of muscles
2. *Elasticity*—the range of motion of a muscle
3. *Tone*—the strength and condition of a muscle

The following tests will help to determine the posture, elasticity, and tone (PET) of your muscles. The exercises that follow will help create an individual "muscle profile" that will help you to correctly condition, position, and stretch muscles. For each of our three categories we will divide the body into the following parts:

1. Arms
2. Legs
3. Lower back
4. Shoulder, upper back, and neck

EXERCISE 1

To determine the *tone* of each body part:
1. Lie on your back with your arms at your sides and the backs of your legs as flat on the floor as possible.
2. "Feel" which of your muscles are relaxed and loose and which are tight and in spasm. Take an inventory as follows:
   1. *Arms*—your biceps in the front of your arm and triceps group in the back, your extensors on the back of the forearm and your flexors in the front.
   2. *Legs*—your biceps in the back of the leg and quadriceps in the front, and your calf muscles.
   3. *Lower back*—the paravertebral muscles, two ropelike muscle groups on either sides of your vertebral column.
   4. *Upper back and neck*—neck muscles, shoulders, muscles between your shoulders.

Your muscles should be relaxed with normal tone. Your shoulders should not be hunched and there should be no uncomfortable feeling of spasm in any muscles. Take the inventory and record your findings below.

PET Profile: Tension		
Muscles	Loose	Tight
Arm — Biceps		
Triceps		
Extensors		
Flexors		
Leg — Biceps		
Quadriceps		
Calf		
Lower Back — Paravertebral		
Upper Back — Neck		
Shoulders		

Fill in your PET Profile.

To determine the range of motion or *elasticity* of each muscle group, one must measure how far the corresponding body part can move. Most restriction of motion is due to poor elasticity of muscles.

EXERCISE 2

Testing the range of your body parts.
1. Arms. Your arms should be able to rotate a half circle (180
   degrees). Raise one arm above your head and then circle it
   down in front of your body. Then try the other one.

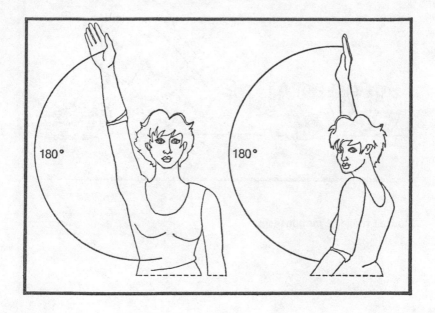

Normal range of motion: arms.

2. Legs. When you are lying down your legs should be able to bend at the hip as shown and your knees should bend 150 degrees.

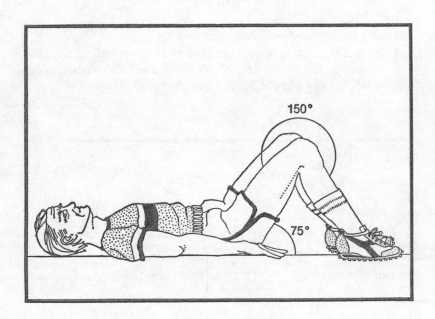

Normal range of motion: legs.

3. Lower back. When standing you should be able to bend at the waist at a 90 degree angle. When standing straight you should be able to plant your feet and swivel your body to the left and right at the waist 90 degrees in each direction. You should be able to arch backward 15 to 20 degrees.

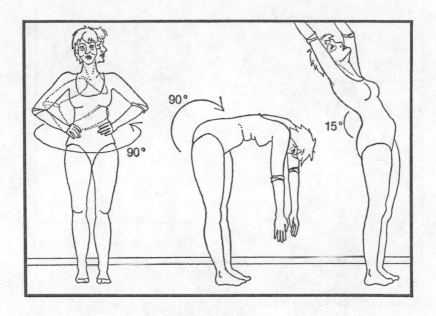

Normal range of motion: back.

4. Shoulder, upper back, and neck. Your head should be able to swivel to the right and to the left 90 degrees, and you should be able to touch your chin to your chest.

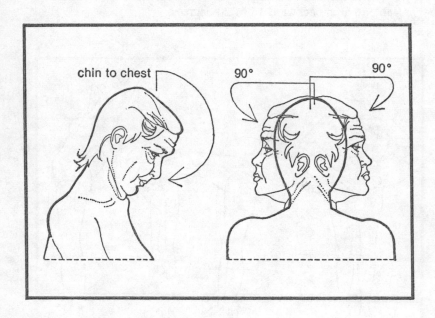

Normal range of motion: neck.

PET Profile: Elasticity		
	Mine	Normal
Arms		
Sideways R		180°
Sideways L		180°
Forward R		180°
Forward L		180°
Hip Bend		
R		75°
L		75°
Knee Bend		
R		150°
L		150°
Waist		
Flex		90°
Extend		15°
Swivel R		90°
Swivel L		90°
Neck		
Chin Touch		to chest
Swivel R		90°
Swivel L		90°

Fill in your Elasticity Profile.

EXERCISE 3

Posture or positioning.
A mirror is required for this exercise.
1. Stand sideways in front of the mirror. Your head should be centered directly over your hips. The small of your back should be curved inward and your neck should also be curved inward. Your shoulders should not be rounded or in a shrugged position, but should be squared with the level of the base of your neck.
2. Stand facing the mirror. Your head should again be centered directly over your hips, not to the side. Your arms should hang loosely and smoothly at your sides. With your heels close but not touching, your feet should point out 2 to 4 inches from an imaginary line drawn between them.

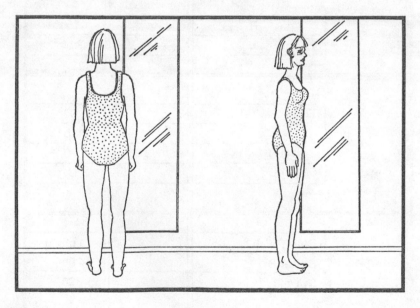

PET Profile: posture.

If you are a typical back pain patient your PET profile (posture, elasticity, and tone) will probably show the following:

Personal PET Profile

The muscles that are tight are:

_____

_____

_____

_____

_____

_____

The joints that swing through an arc
less than normal are:

_____

_____

_____

_____

_____

My posture is poor because of:

Fill in your Personal PET Profile.

TONE — The ropelike muscles on either side of your spine are harder than normal (they are in spasm).

ELASTICITY — You can only bend 15 degrees forward at your waist.

POSTURE — The normally inward curving small of your back is flat and you slouch.

When you have identified your own PET profile, you can begin to work on stretching and toning.

TONE EXERCISE

1. Have your spouse or a friend gently stroke the surface of your skin lightly with the flat of his or her hand for 15 or 20 minutes. The use of a cream or lotion will reduce friction. The surface stroking will gently and over time reduce spasm. After several days you can progress to frictional massage to reduce "binding," but in the early stages stick to gentle stroking.

ELASTICITY EXERCISES

1. Bend your waist to the point where you first feel pain. Do not actively push yourself any further, but allow gravity to gently pull you down another 10 degrees today.
2. Swivel at the waist and allow your momentum to carry you 10 degrees past your initial pain point.
3. If your problem is in your neck, do the same with drooping your head. Remember to always allow gravity and momentum to do the work for you; it is easier and safer.

POSTURE EXERCISES

1. Using your mirror, make an attempt to center your head over your hips rather than in front or to the side.
2. Try to walk without tilting your pelvis to one side (a method unconsciously used to reduce the pressure on one side of the body). Have your spouse or friend place his or her hands over the wing bones at your waist and make sure the two sides are at the same level.

Extend these PET exercises over several days and weeks to include your arm and leg muscles and joints that are stiff. Remember, move up to tolerance, and then only 10 degrees more. *Don't strain.*

In addition to the PET exercises, some familiar, everyday exercises to lengthen and strengthen muscles are important. Tight muscles must slowly be stretched out and weak muscles gradually strengthened. Remember, though, that *gradual* exercise is the key, and that these exercises are not to be done in cases of acute pain, or damage to already acutely inflamed muscles may result. If in doubt, see your doctor.

SIT-UPS

Begin your sit-ups with knees in a bent position, as shown in the illustration. Although bending your knees increases the strain in the abdominal muscles, it decreases the initial tension on the back muscles. Begin with five sit-ups twice a day, and progress to ten and then fifteen twice a day. This exercise will strengthen the abdominal muscles and gradually lengthen the back muscles, which extend from the neck down over the buttocks. If you begin to experience spasm or increasing amounts of pain, *stop,* as overdoing it can cause overlengthened muscles to go into spasm. Do this gently and slowly and build up gradually, and your back muscles will improve in tone over time.

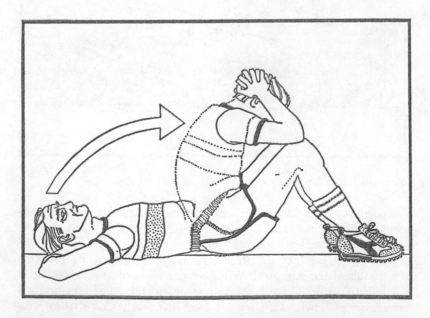

Correct sit-up form.

WILLIAMS' EXTENSION EXERCISE

While the sit-up is designed to strengthen the abdominal muscles and *lengthen* the back muscles, this exercise is designed to actively strengthen, rather than stretch, your back muscles. Lie flat on the floor. Then gently arch your back just off the floor. Again, do this to tolerance and build up over several days or weeks. Generally, you can begin with five repeats twice a day. Proceed to ten and then to fifteen twice a day. Try to hold the arched position for two seconds. If you experience spasm for a day or two in your back muscles, don't panic. It's normal. Any further episodes of spasm, however, should be brought to the attention of your physician immediately.

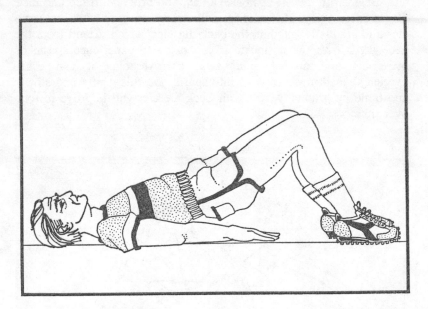

Williams' Extension.

Remember that the sit-up and Williams' exercise are complementary opposites. The sit-up strengthens your abdominal muscles and slowly stretches your back muscles. If done correctly, it increases the strength of the front strut of your spine while reducing the spasms of the rear strut. Williams' exercise does the opposite: it strengthens the rear strut of your spine, mainly the paravertebral muscles, and slowly stretches the front strut of your vertebral column, preventing spasm.

QUADRICEPS STRENGTHENING EXERCISES

The quadriceps is the largest muscle in the body. It is composed of four groups of large muscles in the front and on the inside of the thigh. For the most part, these muscles start above the hip and end in a tendon that is attached to your leg bone, or tibia, just below your knee and which includes in it the knee cap. (The knee cap is called a sesamoid bone, which means that it is a bone which is imbedded in a tendon.) The quadriceps and its tendon give the knee the mechanical advantage necessary to strengthen your leg when it is supporting weight in a fixed position on the ground. This is important for standing and walking. When your muscles are weak, because of disuse, then you will find that your knee buckles and that you pitch forward when you try to walk. Quadriceps exercises are done in a sitting position with your hip and knee bent at 90 degrees. The lower leg, as opposed to the thigh, is then raised to a straight position. Usually you can start with five of these, two or three times a day, and progress over several weeks to ten, ten times a day. Eventually you can put a one- or two-pound weight on your foot (check with your doctor first) and this will help further strengthen the quadriceps muscles.

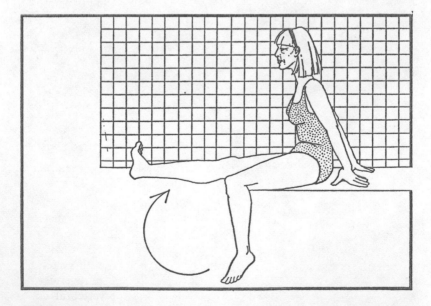

Leg-lift form.

With the PET exercises and the three exercises described above you will be able to strengthen and stretch the muscles that help support your body, and thereby decrease the pain of long-term, chronic disease. You will be able to correct postural and elastic problems in these muscles, and by a process of active conditioning, ensure that your muscles and joints are in the best possible condition to prevent the continuance of chronic pain.

Chapter 17

NIGHTTIME WORRIES: SLEEP AND SEX

Although the problems of pain are pervasive, two major complaints we hear constantly are "I can't sleep, Doctor, the pain keeps me up all night" and, usually mumbled sheepishly into the lapel: "I'm having trouble having . . . you know . . . well, with my wife . . . I'm just not able to do what I used to in bed . . . you know . . . because of the pain." These two issues cause more consternation, dismay, and frustration than any other problems confronted by the chronic pain sufferer. We try to devise simple and practical means to change behavior to fit altered body patterns.

SLEEP

"Sleeping is no mean art: for its sake one must stay awake all day."
NIETZSCHE

You lie awake at night, trying to will yourself to sleep, caught between the day's pulse and the night's peace. Frustration builds as you try to find a comfortable position. Your mind begs for rest; your body aches for relief. It seems as if everyone else is asleep, as if you, in the whole world, are the only one unable to find rest in slumber. It is the time to feel abandoned and alone. Frustration builds as you know that in the morning you will still ache but will have been deprived of a balm that heals. You get up and try to do something productive, to write a letter or read a book, but you are too tired and frustrated to write or read. So you just sit for a while and think, and ache until you again lie down and try to grab hold of elusive rest. The cycle persists until, awakened from a fitful, tossing sleep by the sound of traffic, you know the day must begin and you are not prepared to face it.

This process is repeated over and over in millions of homes. It has been estimated that between 15 and 20 percent of our adult population suffer from some type of insomnia, and among people suffering from chronic pain the percentage is much higher. Sleep deprivation may be the result of multiple or prolonged arousals, difficulty falling asleep, early morning awakening, or poor fitful sleep that does nothing to help rest us. Nonrestorative sleep, in fact, the type we describe above, causes muscle aching, stiffness, nervousness, and irritability, thus perpetuating and intensifying many of the problems of the chronic pain victim.

Sleep research has shown that we pass through five stages during a night's sleep. These are labeled stages one through four, and REM, or Rapid Eye Movement. Stages one through four are often called non-REM sleep. REM sleep is necessary for restorative sleep.

REM sleep was first researched in 1953, and was so named because scientists found that during this stage, which seemed to occur every ninety minutes, a person's eyes were active and roaming in a quick, searching way as if some activity requiring observation were going on. Indeed, it was later discovered that much activity is occurring, for REM sleep is dream sleep. During stages one to four we do not dream and we usually lie still. Every ninety minutes, though, REM sleep occurs and we are able to dream. REM is often accompanied by thrashing and tossing as if in response to activity during the dream.

The sleep cycle is entered at stage one, a light, non-restorative sleep (sleep that does not create a feeling of being rested). If we pass through REM, which normally occurs three or four times during the night, and through stages two and three, we achieve mental and physical relaxation. If we are prevented from dreaming, we awaken unrefreshed and achy. A normal night's sleep might be represented by the graph on the next page.

Pain often prevents REM and stage three sleep from occurring and shortens it by keeping us in a light stage one or two. It is this pattern that prevents us from getting the rest needed to confront the next day. Insomnia is the interruption of the normal sleep cycle.

Each person has a specific sleep requirement and an individual sleep profile (a unique pattern for sleeping). Remember, not everyone requires the same amount of sleep; there is nothing magical about "getting a full eight hours." (In fact, as we age, the amount of

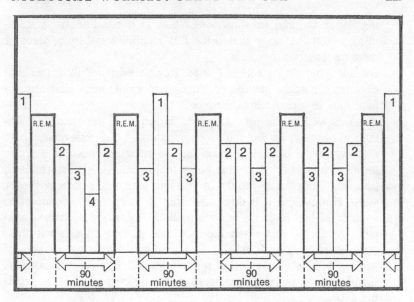

Sleep graph.

sleep we actually need decreases.) What is important is feeling calm, relaxed, and well rested when you waken. In general, the following recommendations should help to build a more normal sleep pattern as well as one that will encourage maximum restorative sleep.

- Autosuggestion helps to set a positive attitude. Even the phrase "I will fall asleep," repeatedly thought or spoken softly, seems to be able to smooth the transition from wakefulness to sleep. It may be simply the repetition that is helpful. Whatever it is, if it works, use it.
- If you have difficulty falling asleep, decrease the number of hours of sleep you get by waking one hour earlier. This may seem counterproductive, but after three or four days it may increase your ability to fall asleep when you first go to bed.
- Change the time you go to sleep. This alters the body's internal clock. If your desire-to-sleep cycle is not in sync with your biological clock, resetting the clock may help.
- Develop a presleep ritual. If you have one thing you can always do before bed, add four more things to it. This may involve read-

ing, letter writing, or showering. This is a conditioning mechanism to tell the body that once this routine has begun, sleep is soon to come.

- Exercise, but do so before 6 P.M. Recent evidence indicates that exercise can stimulate the production of epinephrine and norepinephrine in the brain (chemicals that are depleted in depression) as well as the production of endorphins, the chemical substances thought to be the body's natural pain relievers. There may well be a biological basis for the relaxing effect of exercise on mind and body. Exercise helps to prevent sleep disturbances, tires the body, and builds up certain chemicals necessary for sleep. However, if it is done too close to sleep time, it can act to counter sleep. Exercise may stimulate before it sedates (late-night tennis players often have trouble getting to sleep if their game is after 8 or 9 P.M.). One problem with this method of dealing with insomnia is that many pain sufferers cannot motivate themselves to exercise because they are depressed. Clearly, treating depression will help resolve pain.

- It has recently been discovered that high levels of the brain chemical serotonin are important in promoting sleep. Serotonin, while not present in our daily diet, can be metabolized from tryptophan, an amino acid found in many foods. Many clinicians feel that foods containing tryptophan might help sleep. These include Cheddar cheese, eggs, whole milk, roast beef, ham, hamburgers, and nuts. Tryptophan is also available in drugstores and health-food stores. Some physicians recommend a tablet each night to help induce sleep. It is interesting to note that the level of serotonin in the brain has been shown to be decreased in depressive states. Since chronic pain and depression are linked and both involve a loss of sleep, serotonin may very well play a part in the association between sleeplessness, pain, and depression. In addition, a decrease in the body's response to continued pain stimuli seems to be associated with increased brain serotonin. It is hoped that this field of research will continue to yield tangible results to help combat pain, depression, and insomnia.

- Do not be a sleep stealer. If you sleep during the day, you are robbing yourself of sleep during the night. Many people who complain of sleeplessness at night actually sleep for short bursts during the day; the total *amount* of sleep they get is perfectly adequate. They complain of not being able to sleep simply because they are sleeping less at night.

- Do not stay in bed for anything else but sleep and sex. Try to mentally associate going to bed with falling asleep.
- If you awaken or cannot get to sleep for twenty minutes, get out of bed and listen to easy music, read something dull, even try counting sheep—anything that may help lure you to sleep; but do not do anything interesting to stimulate your body or your mind.
- Finally, a word on one of the most-prescribed medications in the modern pharmacy—the sleeping pill. The regular use of sleeping pills (hypnotics) inhibits their effectiveness. Sleeping pills were not designed to be used on a nightly basis. They will simply stop working. While sleeping pills can help you fall asleep and stay asleep, they do not produce "natural sleep." Almost all sleeping medications reduce the amount of restorative REM sleep. Nonetheless, the overall benefit of using medication for short periods may be positive, especially during times of severe strain. Remember, however, they are to be used on a short-term basis—a few nights to a few weeks at a time. When you expect to have the most difficulty falling and staying asleep, the thought of getting some chemical aid to help you may be soothing in itself. Times when pill use might be appropriate could include a flare-up in your pain, a change in environment, in acute situational stress, or during some modification in your treatment program. Do not hesitate to use them if you need them, but first make certain that you need them.

SEX AND PAIN

Many pain patients have unsatisfying sex lives. Like sleep, a satisfactory sexual life is usually necessary to a sense of fulfillment. Often people with other problems are able to forgo a satisfactory sexual life if they are able to compensate by throwing their efforts into other endeavors, most often work. The patient in pain, however, is cut off from other outlets, which causes further frustration.

Conservatively, one half of our patients with chronic pain have some type of sexual problem. Although initially reluctant to discuss their difficulties, most people open up and are relieved to have professional assistance. Most common are complaints of decreased frequency, painful intercourse, or, intercourse that is compromised by greatly restricted movement. Many pain patients fear their spouse will leave them because they cannot be adequate partners.

Joan Fagin, an attractive forty-year-old, had chronic back pain for four years. She worked sporadically, as husband and three children came first. She cared for their needs as best she could. Sexual activity occurred often but it was a chore and the pain made her wish secretly that she did not have to participate. She felt, however, that she could not tell this to her husband for fear that he would leave and find someone else. Each time he initiated, she tensed for "the pain," but never said "no." Unable to move gracefully, she began to worry that her husband would find her unacceptable and would leave anyway. She could not win. Either guilty or fearful, she spent her nights afraid, unable to sleep, and depressed.

This history is quite typical. A study of the problem was conducted at the Pain Management Center at the Mayo Clinic. In a study of 66 patients, fully two thirds reported a significant deterioration in sexual adjustment, and one third a deterioration of the marriage itself.

There are many reasons why pain interferes with sexual arousal.

1. *Diminished sexual arousal.* Pain itself is a stimulus that decreases sexual arousal. Its presence is distracting and tends to interfere with and override any pleasurable sensation.
2. *Fear.* The fear of pain during intercourse can decrease or turn off sexual arousal completely.
3. *Lack of muscle tone.* Unused, the muscles hurt. When people avoid using muscles in any type of exercise and then begin to use them, there is a stiffness and soreness which increases the level of pain already present.
4. *Worry about further damage.* The illusion that the pain means that there is continued and further damage to muscles, ligaments, and joints often prevents people not only from having a fulfilling sexual encounter, but from doing many other jobs and engaging in other pleasures.
5. *Distancing from partner.* Pain is a distancer. It provokes alienation and isolation. This distancing, of course, can destroy the intimacy needed for sexual encounters.
6. *Medication.* Many of the medications used for the treatment of pain carry with them the side effects of drowsiness, lethargy, and decreased sexual interest.
7. *Depression.* The depression that often accompanies pain has as one of its cardinal symptoms a decrease in libido.

A first step in helping to solve sexual problems is speaking about them. Many pain patients deprive themselves of the chance to openly discuss their fears, discomforts, or anxieties with their spouses, doctors, or others who may be able to help. Speaking openly may prevent or alleviate a sense of guilt or worry, which, unchecked, can build to the point where it, too, interferes with sex.

When it is difficult to move spontaneously or to lie in one position, other means of sexual enjoyment are possible. Many pain patients cannot maneuver sufficiently without pain to enjoy coitus, but noncoital methods of intimacy are available. Manual and oral sex can be used to satisfy both partners. If coitus is attempted, the position which is the least painful to either partner with pain usually involves the male in back of the woman, both on their sides nestled spoon fashion. The muscles are least stressed in this position and can be used for greater lengths of time. Finally, the Masters and Johnson method of sensate focus, involving gentle touching and stroking in comfortable positions, is often pain-free and satisfying. There are many excellent, well-illustrated "sex manuals" currently available. Research and experimentation may help solve some vexing problems.

Sex need not be the worry-fraught ordeal it seems to be for many pain patients. With open discussion, mutual planning, and plenty of understanding, a satisfactory sexual adaptation to pain can be achieved. Don't be timid. Sexual relations are an important aspect of a couple's life together. Open up and seek some new solutions.

Chapter 18

CREATING THE PAIN DIARY

Close your eyes and try to picture this scene. You're sitting at the end of an examining table in your doctor's office. The nurse has left you a giant paper towel, optimistically called a disposable gown, to put on in preparation for the "visit." He has not yet arrived. You hear his voice, through the walls, down the halls. He is talking to someone else. It sounds like he's busy, something about a patient in the cardiac care unit. He asks his nurse, "Who is waiting?" Doors slam. He sounds busy, also a little angry.

The room you're in is sterile; it's also freezing. The paper gown is not warm. You feel silly. The perspiration pours off as if someone had turned a faucet on in your armpits. The only distraction is a rubber reflex hammer which is chained to the wall. You tap nervously on your knee, connecting every third time with a reflex circuit causing your leg to kick out automatically. You work!

It's now been 10 minutes of waiting. The draft is incredible; your breath mists. One moment, you consider leaving, the next, crying. You decide to wait. You think you're angry, but are too frightened to admit it.

Finally he comes, greets you by name, and asks how you're doing while he begins the laying on of hands.

You tell him you are cold, and, of course, that you still hurt.

He stops his exam, looks you in the eye, and says, "Is the pain any worse?"

"Oh, yes, I feel terrible this morning."

Stop. The idea that any sane person could under these conditions present an accurate record of his therapeutic progress, or lack thereof, is ridiculous. The presentation of an accurate history, which is essential to the treatment of chronic pain, requires a far more creative and reflective process.

We take it for granted that important information simply flows out of you when you walk into a doctor's office. This is hardly the case. The following resistances can grossly interfere with an accurate history.

1. You are too cold to talk.
2. Memories are selective. In looking back at an event or illness, we recall certain aspects—perhaps the most painful or pleasant —and selectively overvalue their importance. We remember *moments,* not days or weeks.
3. Visiting a doctor is a stressful experience. The examining-room scene described above is not uncommon. It's easy to become frightened or intimidated.
4. A lot of what you remember to say depends on your mood. Although it may be months between visits, you're going to report what's most important on the day of your visit. If it's a good day, then you may be less attentive to problems that you had two weeks before.
5. Conversely, if you are feeling poorly, the report may be unduly negative or discouraging. *Moods change rapidly, pain conditions don't.*
6. The doctor has only a limited time to spend with you and may focus on an issue he feels is important. How do you get him to pay attention to *your* priorities?

The problem of trying to keep everything in mind is a bit like juggling a dozen items at once. Somehow, there must be a better way.

A NEED FOR ACCURATE RECORDS

To help our patients keep straight everything they have to know, we tried an experiment: we ordered notebooks for them with the words "Pain Management Program" imprinted in gold letters. We encouraged people to write things down as they happened, to record as much of the proceedings as they could. Our goal was to create a sense of involvement—to absorb people into the program.

The experiment worked well; having notes helped. Patients would, without any direction, use their notebooks to record observations, questions, and ideas that came to them in the time between sessions.

Gradually the teaching sessions became more fruitful. Questions were more specific and more accurately reflected the individual's problems. Subjective reports of which activities and behavior made pain better or worse were more precise. People could actually see in black and white what helped and what did not. We were overjoyed. Most fortuitously, we had stumbled upon an important therapeutic tool—the personal pain record.

The "pain diary" is the simplest and most efficient way to detail the specifics of what could be a very vague and subjective subject— your pain. Maintaining a detailed record of pain, in the course of treatment, ultimately makes you a collaborator in your own treatment, breaking you out of the role of the "patient-object."

What To Do

In Appendix A you will find a copy of the thirty-day pain diary for your personal use. The directions are fairly simple, intentionally so. If the process were too arduous, no one would do it. Nonetheless, completing the record accurately will require a little concentration and persistence.

The completion of the pain diary begins with the recording of the pain experience. We recommend that you begin the recording of information *thirty days before your next doctor's visit*. All directions are in the form of a countdown beginning at day thirty and counting down to "D-day," or doctor's visit.

The first step may be to make an appointment with your doctor. We are not trying to drum up business for America's physicians. Quite the contrary, our intention is to help you get more valuable direction out of your physician's office visit. Our assumption is that you will make some routine visits anyway. While it would be presumptuous to try to outsmart or arbitrarily contest the judgment of your family physician, what you must do, and do quite well, is know a great deal about your pain. The diary is an objective visible record of the past thirty days' problems, an accurate and complete record of your difficulties, one that avoids the pitfalls of vague, inconsequential statements such as "My back still hurts" or "I have not gotten any better."

Work on your personal pain diary for the next thirty days. We are absolutely certain that the value of accurate record keeping will be apparent.

Rating Pain

Pain rating is a one-to-ten scoring system for measuring the amount of pain you are feeling at selected times during the course of the day. The pain rating scale below correlates a number value with the description of pain states.

PAIN RATING SCALE

0   *No pain.*

1–3. *Mild pain*—While quite noticeable, does not interfere with the usual daily activity.

4–6. *Moderate pain*—Causing curtailment of daily activities and physical sense of distress.

7–8. *Moderately severe pain*—Causing major problems in function and intense discomfort.

9.   *Severe pain*—No functioning possible. Unbearable discomfort.

10.   *Most severe pain imaginable.*

EXAMPLE:

Joe Smith awakes. He feels stiff as a board. Lying quietly in bed, he focuses his attention on an area of his lower back that is the center of his pain. Although stiff and sleepy, he notes that there is local tenderness, but no really severe radiation of pain down his legs. Joe assesses his pain as 4 (moderate) this morning. Taking his pain diary, he records his morning pain as a four.

Joe gets up, dresses, eats breakfast, and leaves for work. He spends the morning uncomfortably, breaks for lunch, then attends a staff meeting. Being engaged in a stimulating discussion over a proposed new project, Joe hardly notices his back pain. Following the meeting, he feels invigorated, having achieved concessions which enhance his managerial responsibility. He feels minor pain, but does not think it interferes with his activities. He rates his pain as a two.

Driving home after work, he gets caught in traffic. The delay is tedious. After such an "up" day, sitting behind the wheel makes him acutely aware of his back. The driver's seat of his seven-year-old Chevy station wagon, a car he would love to trade but cannot afford to, offers minimal support for his lower back. When he finally arrives home, late for dinner, his wife is furious. Their beautiful prime roast

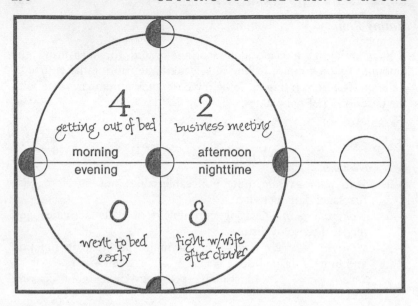

Sample pain rating scale.

is beyond well done. She tells him he could have at least phoned. Joe explains himself. Frustrated, he eats his overcooked, dried roast beef.

Sitting down on the sofa after dinner, he is informed that his twelve-year-old son, Randy, has been suspended from school for one day for writing obscene graffiti in the hall outside the principal's office. Joe is enraged. He scolds Randy. Randy pouts and accuses his dad of taking out his frustrations on him. "Just because you don't feel well, do you have to be so mean to me?" Randy alleges his dad is incapable of understanding the needs of a twelve-year-old; he finds his father insensitive. Joe is discouraged. His back aches so intensely he can no longer sit on the couch. He retreats to his bedroom and rates his pain as an eight.

Before retiring, he ingests three aspirin and 10 milligrams of Valium. Without much difficulty, he falls asleep, and sensing the regressive comfort of a good night's rest, lies comfortably till morning. *No* pain rating.

In Appendix A, you will find several pages on which to record the intensity of your pain. Beginning at day thirty, and then at five-day intervals thereafter, record the pain experience four times during the course of the day: morning, afternoon, evening, and night (if you happen to be up and in pain). At the end of thirty days you will have six "randomly selected" days to analyze. For each pain rating, record the activity you were involved in *just prior to making the pain rating*. A word or two will suffice.

OBSERVATIONS OF OTHER PAIN RATERS

Learning to subjectively rate pain serves several functions. The following list of observations is condensed from other patients' experiences. Have you discovered any similarities?

1. "Small changes in my mood can greatly affect how much I notice my pain."

2. "The whole idea of having to again score the pain has helped me to focus. . . . It is really not always the same. . . . It does change from day to day."

3. "I was amazed to see how much anger affected my pain. It doubled in intensity whenever I fought with my spouse or got angry with the kids."

4. "What really pleased me was losing ten pounds last month; I am not sure it made the pain any better, though."

5. "I thought the whole thing was silly, but it made me think about what was happening in my body. Learning relaxation also helped; my pain really went down during the month."

6. "Evenings were a real trigger for my back. It is amazing how little I felt my pain during the day, but once I got home, it was terrible."

7. "After I finished the diary, I was surprised. For some reason I believed my neck hurt worse sitting at my desk in the office. In fact, I complained specifically about the problem to my doctor on many occasions. My record just does not bear that out. Half the time I was too busy (and probably not very focused on my pain) to make a rating. I was surprised that the morning pain rating was so high. I must have an anticipatory pain; it goes away when I get to work."

8. "There was no correlation between anything I did and my pain. I found no consistency. Sometimes it was better in the morning, sometimes worse."

9. "I was amazed at how rapidly my pain became intolerable. I would be fine in the morning and then wham! It would hit me like a lightning bolt."

10. "Initially, getting out for walks made me feel worse the next
day. But I persisted and by the end of the month I was walking five blocks. This was much more than I had ever been
able to do before."

COMMENTS

For years we have relied on the pain complaint to assess the therapeutic process of a patient. Is pain really the whole story? Probably
not. It is quite clear that people "feel better" and truly get better without much change in their pain complaint. Looking at the patient observations, we found that many people simply did not notice much
change. Their pain was rigid and fixed, while others reported feeling
"better" with no change in the pain state. However, the majority
identified activities that either helped or hurt. In most cases, pain
waxed and waned in response to certain sets of conditions. Identifying *the pain enhancers and pain reducers* is the next step in their
diary record.

Pain Enhancers and Pain Reducers

Is there a connection between how you spend your time and the
amount of pain you experience? Do certain activities make you feel
better, others worse? The first step in answering the question may be
to detail how you actually spend your time.

CONCEPT OF AN ACTIVITY RECORD

Frequently, when we ask a patient how he spends his time, the response is vague and nonspecific, and of little help to us. Responses
like "I don't do anything—I stay at home," "I rest during the day.
I'm in too much pain to do anything that requires too much effort,"
"Exercise makes my pain worse," and "Nothing much" are common. The reason is simple. Slowly and almost imperceptibly,
chronic pain has destroyed the structure, the timetable, of a person's
life. Structure is responsible for creating priorities and maintaining
schedules. Being responsible for various activities provides a framework for a person's life. The sense of personal well-being and vocational adequacy one seeks is often a function of doing a job in an
organized and structured manner. Being out of work, staying up all
night pacing the floor, and eating to suppress anxiety or relieve boredom are *effects* of chronic pain that serve to disrupt the organization

WHEN	WHAT	WHERE	WITH WHOM	PAIN BETTER	PAIN WORSE
First awakening	EAT BREAKFAST	KITCHEN	CHILDREN		X
Mid-morning	READ PAPER	KITCHEN	ALONE	X	
Noon	LUNCH/READ MAIL	KITCHEN	ALONE	X	
Afternoon	WATCHING TV	LIVING ROOM	ALONE		X
Evening	WATCHING TV	LIVING ROOM	WIFE & KIDS	X	
Nighttime	PACING	UPSTAIRS	ALONE		X

Sample daily activity record.

of a person's day, ruining an individual's confidence and lowering self-esteem. The physical and emotional consequences can be devastating. Chronic fatigue, mounting depression, muscular tension, and chronic anxiety are but a few of the many possible problems resulting from the loss of a daily structure.

COMPLETING A WORKSHEET

In the Pain Diary there are a number of blank worksheets entitled "Daily Record." The concept is simple. You are asked to record your activity at selected times during the day, as well as, where you were, who you were with, and whether the pain was better or worse. We suggest that you record this information on days 30, 25, 20, 15, and 10, as you count down to your physician's office visit. A sample daily record is included for illustration. (Note: The daily record is completed at five-day intervals as a matter of convenience. The random sampling will generally present a fairly representative picture of your regular activities.)

Upon completing the final daily record, five days before your office visit, analyze the results. The following questions are designed to help organize the activity information:

1. What is the most common activity?
2. Do you tend to be in *one* place most of the day?
3. There are six points during the day when you are asked to check your activity. On the average, how many times are you alone?
4. Are certain activities associated with increased pain? If so, these activities can be considered *pain enhancers*. List them.
5. Are there certain activities associated with decreased pain? If so, these activities can be considered *pain reducers*. List them.

FOR THE TRULY AMBITIOUS

If you truly enjoy record keeping, this next table will prove a joy. It's not essential, but if you want to have a more detailed record of your pain enhancers and reducers, you can proceed.

In the pain diary there is a "pain tolerance" table. The day's activities are divided into "activities" and "passivities." This table should be completed once, based upon an "average day" during the course of the month. Next to each item you are asked to record the *approximate* number of hours of each day spent performing each activity. Then record your subjective pain rating.

As there are ten "activities" and ten "passivities," the totals divided by ten will give you the average pain rating for all activity (and all passivity). Select the most severe *enhancers* from "activities" and "passivities," and list them below the pain tolerance table in the spaces provided. Now find the three items with the lowest rating. List them as pain reducers.

RECOGNIZING DRUG EFFECT

In Chapter 13, we describe the major classes of medications used in the treatment of pain. Most people with pain take many different medications. Everyone who uses a medicine should be aware of the side effects and positive benefits of that medication as well as the specific reasons for taking it. As a patient taking a medication, you are the best judge of how effective a particular drug is in controlling your pain.

The drug effect chart asks you to list all of the medications you are currently using, the reasons (as you understand them) for their use, and the positive and negative effects of the drug. A sample drug effect table is shown. In the diary, list all the drugs you are presently using and how you believe they are affecting you. Be certain to bring this table with you on your next visit to discuss these observations with your physician.

People react differently to various medications. For example, some people find Valium is a great help, while others are overly sedated by this medication. Codeine, an excellent analgesic for some, gives others incredible headaches and upset stomachs. There are a host of individual responses to even the mildest medication. Knowing in detail how you respond to a particular drug will help your physician prescribe more effectively and ultimately provide you with the single best medication for your problem.

MEDICATION RECORD KEEPING

How much medication are you actually taking? If the directions on the bottle say three or four times per day, are you following those instructions?

Actually, very few people follow physicians' directions when it comes to using medications. In some studies of general medical pa-

Name of Medicine	Reason for Use	Drug Effect Positive	Drug Effect Negative
1 Aspirin	•pain relief	• dulls pain	•upset stomach
2 Percodan	•very bad pain	• sometimes reduces sharpness of pain	• nausea ◦ changes in mood
3 Motrin	• not sure	•helps my arthritis	•upset stomach

Sample drug effect table.

tients, as few as 10 percent of people actually use the medication as prescribed. Many people never even fill the doctor's prescription or, if they do, simply file the bottle neatly away in the medicine cabinet for future reference. Worst of all are those whimsical people who gobble pills when they feel the need and ignore directions when they feel better. All of us, at one time or another, simply forget, missing doses for hours, even days, at a time.

It is very difficult to determine the effectiveness of a drug when the dosage and ingestion of the medication is varied by chance. As we have detailed in Chapter 13, many factors can influence the potential effect of a drug. An accurate record of how much and how often you use a medication can only help minimize "drug variability" and help figure out what helps and what does not.

In the diary, you will find some "one-week medication records." As many people with chronic pain take medication for extended periods, use the table to compare medication use at various times during the course of the next several months.

Name of Medicine		Day 1			
		M	A	E	N
1	Aspirin	4	4	2	
2	Motrin	1		1	1
3	Percodan	2		1	
	Tylenol with Codeine				
4	Valium	1	1	1	1
5	Seconal				2

Sample day of weekly medication record. (M=morning, A=afternoon, E=evening, N=nighttime.)

In a given week how regularly do you use your medications? Are there some medications you are more likely to forget? Are there drugs you tend to use excessively?

Over time, if you keep medication records (one effective method would be to fill out the table on the last week of every month), you will have an ongoing record of your drug-use trend. This record will help you to answer the following questions:

1. As your therapy progresses are you using less medication?
2. Are you developing patterns of abuse?
3. Are you taking more narcotics or less?
4. Do you require more potent pain relievers or milder agents?
5. Have new problems emerged that require new therapies?

There may be other questions that you have, especially if you keep an accurate record to detail your progress.

The medication you are using can create serious problems, especially if irregular, inappropriate, inadequate, or excessive patterns of use develop. Be particular, take notes, keep records. To summarize, a medication journal is useful:

1. To provide an accurate record of medication.

2. For analysis of actual drug effects.
3. As a basis for reevaluation of usefulness and effectiveness of each medication.
4. To achieve greater pain control through more appropriate use of medication.
5. For early detection of abuse problems.

COMMENTS

In the diary is space for comments. Record any private thoughts you might want to discuss at some later time with your physician regarding the use of medication.

RELAXATION RATING

Chapter 15 outlines the concept of progressive relaxation as a method for pain control. The diary provides an opportunity to chart your progress beginning on day 30 and then counting down to 25, 20, 15, 10, 5—so six days of relaxation ratings will be recorded.

Each day record your relaxation level in the morning, afternoon, and evening, after you've practiced your progressive relaxation exercises. Record the "relaxation rating" in the appropriate time segment.

RELAXATION LEVELS

0   Unbearable tension.
1–3.   Severe agitation associated with mental irritability. Motor activity characterized by pacing, sweating, and severe muscle spasm.
4–6.   Moderate agitation. Generalized internal feeling of *unrest* without outward signs. High levels of inner tension.
7–8.   A sense of inner relief while still slightly tense. A beginning sense of being in control.
9.   A definite sense of calmness and relaxation, although awareness of problems is still present. A sense of relative ease.
10.   Total, complete relaxation. Freedom from body tension.

ON DIARIES

We have limited our diary to a few critical items including pain rating, medication use, activity charting, and relaxation rating. By simplifying the method we hope to produce a concise, pragmatic record that can aid you in your quest for medical treatment. By augmenting your record keeping skills, you can become a more accurate historian able to identify therapeutic trends and patterns or responses at early stages. Early intervention can forestall crisis and prevent disability. Sometimes doing little things at the appropriate moments prevents the need to implement massive measures when the problem gets out of hand. It was all said long ago. Something about a stitch in time . . .

Chapter 19

HELPFUL HINTS

HELPFUL HINT NO. 1: Always Break Up Tasks into Small, Manageable Bits

There is nothing more encouraging than success. Whether we are talking about a five-hundred-piece jigsaw puzzle or the management of pain, there is nothing more satisfying than completing what you set out to do and nothing worse than being so overwhelmed that you become paralyzed.

A friend, a sufferer from chronic pain, was feeling somewhat better than usual one fall day. Being ambitious and helpful, he decided that he would show his wife, out of town for a meeting, how much better he was doing by raking all the leaves around his home. This friend, of course, had felt frustrated by not being able to help his wife with the household tasks and felt that here, finally, was a chance to help, to show that he was still capable. Now, as anyone with a tree or two in his yard knows, raking leaves is one of these strange tasks which defy natural physical law. That is, the more you rake, the more leaves appear. My friend decided to rake the whole yard before his wife returned the next day. What a splendid gift it would make for her. It turned out to be a horror. A naturally back-breaking job under any circumstances, it was overwhelming, for a man not used to using his back and arm muscles. Needing to please his wife and show her that he was still able to do his part, he raked and raked and by suppertime he found that fully half the leaves were still there. Obsessed by his desire to finish in one day, he went back out—but was more frustrated and angry when by 9 P.M., fully one quarter of his leaves were still there and he could not move for

stiffness. Pushing on, becoming more overwhelmed. Well, the end of
the story is that he did finish—at midnight. His wife was very
pleased, the yard looked splendid, and my friend spent the next four
weeks in traction, somewhere between agony and purgatory. His
need to reassert his competence in the eyes of his wife had overwhelmed him. He took on too much. He should have determined
what his "manageable bit" was and stuck to it, doing a little each
day. His wife would still have been pleased, the leaves would have
been raked, and he would have been in less pain and not in the hospital. He could have controlled his pain and the next four weeks of
his life by remembering this helpful hint.

HELPFUL HINT NO. 2:   Pain Enhancers and Pain Reducers

Pain enhancers and reducers are referred to elsewhere in this
book. It is, however, worth reinforcing this somewhat obvious equa-
tion: If the things in your life that increase your pain outweigh the
things in your life that reduce your pain, you will experience pain.
And vice versa. It is as obvious a statement as the financial adage
"Buy low, sell high." Most investors, however do just the opposite.
They run with the pack. That is, they sell low and buy high because
they are lost and frightened and do not understand the dynamics of
the stock market. So, too, with pain. People become frightened when
they do not understand, for instance, that pain medication has
stopped working. They begin to imagine that their injury has worsened, rather than understanding that the medicine has stopped
working because their body has become used to it. The fright causes
anxiety, which makes the pain worse, which then provokes the need
for more medicine, which does not work anyway, and so on and so
on. Know what makes your pain worse and what makes your pain
better. In detail. Make a list of both. If vacuuming the drapes causes
shoulder pain but washing the sink does not, avoid one and do the
other. Multiply this by the hundreds of pain reducers and enhancers
that occur in each day's activities and you stand a good chance of
devising a daily plan that includes as many reducers and as few
enhancers as possible.

Charles Dickens, in *David Copperfield,* gives us a parallel definition of poverty and wealth and thus a plan for achieving whichever
of the two we want. "Wealth," said Dickens, "is sixpence in and

fivepence out. Poverty, on the other hand, is fivepence in and six-pence out."

HELPFUL HINT NO. 3:   Pain Is Not Injury

There once was a football coach who earned great regard from his players with the following admonition: "Fellows, to play football, one must be able to distinguish pain from injury."

This is no small distinction. We are products of conditioning. From childhood, we learn that pain means injury. Indeed, in acute pain our pain body is telling us that there is injury and that we had better take care of it—immediately. In chronic pain, though, the injury is over and only the pain lingers on. If one confuses pain and injury, then, like football players who do not learn well, we step out of the game. Chronic pain is not a signal to stop life. It is not a warning that damage is increasing. It is a signal to the prudent: ease up, but never stop playing.

HELPFUL HINT NO. 4:   There Is No Unitary Cure for Chronic Pain

We are once again discovering that illness and disease do not pop up from a single source. Similarly, there is no one cure for any disease. Illness is an amalgam, a mixture of the right germ at the right time plus a genetic predisposition to get certain kinds of problems plus stress plus personality plus a whole host of other environmental, physical, and developmental events. From a strep throat to cancer, we are products of our heritage, our environment, our development, and our personality.

We say that we are only rediscovering this fact, because Plato first enunciated it many thousands of years ago. In the eighteenth century the philosopher René Descartes proposed that mind and body were separate and isolated entities and unaffected by each other. We are just now coming to understand that Plato was correct, not Descartes, and so we can no longer look for unitary cures for our illnesses. Identify as many causes for your pain as you can—physical, emotional, and environmental—but do not expect a single cure or your disappointment may well be another cause for your pain.

HELPFUL HINT NO. 5:   Biological Clocks

Each person has several biological built-in clocks that control his internal cycles. One cycle is through in minutes, another in hours, one in days, and some cycles take years. If you can learn to read these clocks, you can determine when is the best time for certain activities. For instance, if you know that you are strongest at night, save some tasks that require extra strength or concentration for the evening. If you are depressed in the morning, do not attempt complicated or difficult tasks until after lunch.

Learning to read yourself and gearing your activity to biological rhythms is a difficult task. Scientists are just beginning to understand these cycles. In a recent experiment, a lethal dose of *E. coli* bacteria was given to a group of mice at their subjective noon. Eighty-three percent of the mice died. However, when the same bacteria and the same dose were given to the mice at their subjective midnight, only 15 percent died. Why? Was there some immunological mechanism that was stronger at midnight than at noon? We don't know. We do know, however, that the rhythm that controls immunity can also control other functions—including pain. At some time in the future we may be able to control these rhythms. At the present time, you can benefit by being aware of yours.

Chapter 20

FOR THOSE IN PAIN: THE BEST
OF CARE

WHAT IS GOOD TREATMENT?

Based on the newer research that has been described, since 1975 new treatment strategies have been developed in both the physical and the psychological realms of the chronic pain system. In order to understand these new therapies and to best apply them to your situation, let us follow two patients through their journeys from pain suffering to treatment to successful management. These are composite histories which are presented to demonstrate what can be done with combinations of the newer therapy under the proper care of a concerned and competent physician.

Mike was a twenty-eight-year-old electrician, married, with three children. He worked for an electrical contractor. His life was organized and pleasant. He had just bought a new home and his family life was satisfying and rewarding.

In June 1978, Mike fell from a ladder and injured his back. At first he felt pain only in his lower back and, after resting in bed with the heating pad for several days, returned to work. Soon, however, he began to experience increasing amounts of sharp pain and muscle spasm with some radiation of pain down his left leg. More frequent bouts of bed rest and muscle relaxants were required. As Mike was paid only when he worked, his financial condition began to deteriorate. After four months, his physician sent Mike to an orthopedic surgeon, as he was concerned about the longevity of Mike's illness. The surgeon suggested that Mike be hospitalized, placed in traction, and undergo a myelogram to determine whether he had injured a disk. The myelogram was positive. Mike had in fact herniated a disk and surgery was performed in two days' time. The disk was removed and for a short while Mike began to feel better.

His recovery was slow. Four months later Mike began to notice pain again. This time, however, it radiated from his back all the way down his left leg and into his toes. The pain was intermittent but knifelike. He also began to experience a burning sensation in his left leg. Muscle spasms again became a problem and his doctor placed Mike on antispasmodics and Percodan for the pain. The doctor told Mike, however, that the *Percodan could only be a temporary measure* and that he had better start a rehabilitation and physical therapy program aimed at attacking the chronic pain problem. The pain, in all, had lasted two and a half years by this time. Mike was unable to work and had to manage on workmen's compensation. Moreover, he had grown irritable and depressed. His family life had become intolerable, not only to Mike but to his wife and children. It seemed Mike was always in pain and always complaining. Everything was a task for him. The minor chores of cleaning up after meals or helping with the vacuuming or dusting were insurmountable problems that seemed to perpetuate his pain. Mike felt guilty about not being able to participate in the care and upkeep of his home. He took out his frustrations not only on himself but on his family, frequently losing patience with his children and scolding them unnecessarily and harshly. One day his wife threatened to leave. She could not tolerate the constant bickering and screaming. "I promised to love, honor, and obey, but this was ridiculous. He used me as his whipping boy. Every time he had a problem, he blamed me. I know he was frustrated, but he just could not keep taking it out on me." Things had reached crisis proportions and Mike felt overwhelmed and lost. In desperation, he called his family doctor.

Things had gone too far. From a satisfied and well-liked family man and worker, Mike had turned into an irritable, depressed, and pained man who was taking large amounts of medication, was impossible to live with, and felt unproductive and unworthy. He was a victim of a chronic pain syndrome. With the help of his doctor, Mike began to get hold of his life again. The medication that Mike was taking for pain was cut gradually down to a minimal amount. He had been unquestionably abusing the pain-killer and this was affecting his behavior and his psychological well-being. Some family counseling and the use of antidepressant medication helped soothe some rather jangled nerves.

As far as the back spasms were concerned, a new treatment was implemented under his physician's direction. A transcutaneous nerve stimulator (a small, externally worn device which electronically stimulates nerves; see pages 283–84) delivered a weak electrical current to Mike's paraspinal muscles which was designed to "override" the pain of the spasm. His pain began to gradually decrease. When he wore the box, he could be relatively pain-free for a short period.

Repeat surgery was ruled out. After all, it had not helped that much the first time around. In fact, as a result of the surgery he had developed arachnoiditis—an inflammation of the ligamentous covering of the spine. This problem caused as much pain as the original injury. After a prolonged consultation with Mike's doctor, it was felt that the arachnoiditis would likely recur with repeat surgery. The decision not to reoperate was a joint one reached by doctor and patient. It was quite a significant decision, one which required a rather extensive discussion of the potential benefits and risks.

It was felt, however, that the burning in Mike's leg was probably caused by reflex sympathetic dystrophy (a nerve disorder that typically causes a burning sensation pain; see page 63). Additionally, pressure on his sciatic nerve created knifelike pains in his legs. In the hope that it would relieve both the burning and knifelike pains, Mike was given a series of five epidermal injections—or nerve blocks into the spinal canal (the injection of a mixture of long-acting anesthetic agents and cortisone at the roots of the spinal nerves; a procedure which may provide temporary pain reduction). These were effective against both types of pain. Mike began to feel some moderate relief. Over time, the pain-free moments became longer and longer. He was able to do more and more and became physically more active.

As the physical pain problems became less burdensome, more attention could be placed on the psychosocial aspects of his disability. His doctor, pleased with the very positive results of family therapy, suggested that Mike start in a pain group. Just as the family therapy helped to explain the family's role in the perpetuation of the pain syndrome, the pain group would help Mike cope with the stress and disability of being at home, out of work, and consumed in a slow, arduous process of healing. The group did, in fact, help him feel more a part of things. For the first time since he was injured, he felt as if he could learn techniques from other people for dealing with whatever pain remained.

The combination of a transcutaneous nerve stimulator, nerve blocks, medication reduction, antidepressant medication, family group therapy, and pain group participation worked. Mike and his family came to know how his pain syndrome worked almost as well as his doctors. They were able to deal effectively with any limitations it placed on them and they felt freer to express their anger as well as joys with each other. As the pain receded in importance, Mike was again able to go back to work, first on a part-time basis and then full time. He and his family were able to go on with their lives. There were limitations; Mike had to wear the TNS unit sometimes, and he had to restrict certain physical activities. He attended weekly group sessions for a year and he needed physical therapy every two weeks. But these were gladly accepted by the family and Mike. He could now function almost as he had before.

Brenda, thirty-six years old, was a computer science technician. An easygoing person, she seemed eager to please—at times a bit too eager. She was a mite too sugary, a trait that tended to put people off. Although outwardly sweet, always complimenting and praising others, she was underneath an intense and nervous person who needed to be in total control of every situation. Her self-esteem was quite low.

She suffered from chronic unremitting headaches that began at the back of her neck and soon covered her head like a cap. When she had one of these headaches, which occurred every three or four days, Brenda had to go to the nurses' station and lie down for several hours. The pain made it impossible to work.

Brenda was markedly overweight and smoked upwards of two packs of cigarettes a day. She liked warm and smoky rooms, a need which offended many of her coworkers. The headaches were threatening her job. Although she could do an excellent job when she set her mind to it, she was frequently sick or in need of rest. Her supervisor became increasingly disappointed with her performance. She warned Brenda that her job was in jeopardy. Finally, after many months, Brenda sought help. She went to consult her family physician, who set up a program for Brenda which included treatment, not just for the headaches, but for changing the way she dealt with life. This doctor knew Brenda and he could look and see more than just headaches when he examined her. After a thorough neurological work-up, it was decided that Brenda's headaches were of a tension type. Muscle contraction, constant worry, and a tense, controlling attitude helped fuel the problem. The doctor felt she was significantly depressed and that depression was a major cause of the headaches. He referred her to a physician trained to deal with pain syndromes.

Brenda was started on a ten-week course of biofeedback for the treatment of her headaches. She was taught to control the muscle contraction in her neck before she got a headache. A thorough exposure to relaxation training helped break the cycle of anxiety— muscle tension headaches—anxiety.

Brenda was so impressed by her behavioral changes and the decrease in her headaches that she requested additional psychological therapy. A brief course of supportive psychotherapy was offered to help her define her goals and initiate a program for reconsidering the way she dealt with some of the people in her life. It was not long before she recognized that her flowery, overly sweet demeanor was a cover to hide the nervousness she felt in being with people. "I was always too afraid people would not like me, especially if they knew how I really was. I did everything I could to please them. Knowing that I am really not such a bad person certainly helps. I feel much less defensive. It has taken a burden off." Brenda got much better with a little help. It was decided that long-term, ten-years-on-the-couch psychoanalysis was not needed. The brief (twelve-week) once-a-week method had helped others formulate goals and change behavior, and it was equally as helpful to Brenda. In addition, the insight she gained led her to a diet workshop and Smokenders. She felt like a new person and was going to do everything she could to improve her health. Six months later, Brenda was working, rarely missing a day's work because of illness. She had finished her course of therapy. She did not quit smoking entirely, but did cut down to half of her previous cigarette consumption. She lost thirty pounds. She began to mix with friends and started dating once again. For her, the outcome of her pain therapy was successful in more ways than she had ever anticipated.

Fortunately, Brenda and Mike were able to put it all together. Under the skilled direction of competent physicians, all the useful and necessary components of therapy were combined and implemented in an intelligent, comprehensive program. Brenda and Mike were counseled and consulted at every turn to ensure complete participation in their recovery. Each was made a collaborator against the illness. They were totally involved in their treatment.

But not everyone is so fortunate. Finding a skilled, concerned physician who wants to actively include you in the course of your treatment is not a matter of chance. *It is up to you.*

The key to pain control is in taking responsibility for your own treatment, by learning about pain, recognizing the devastating consequences of chronic pain syndromes, and taking an active role in the course of your treatment. For every patient we recommend a personal pain control program, where even the most minor aspect of health care becomes a matter of personal concern. Early intervention and prompt identification of problems can forestall serious complications. Get started today. The best intervention is the one you make now.

APPENDICES

Appendix A

THE PAIN DIARY

Appendix A

RATING PAIN

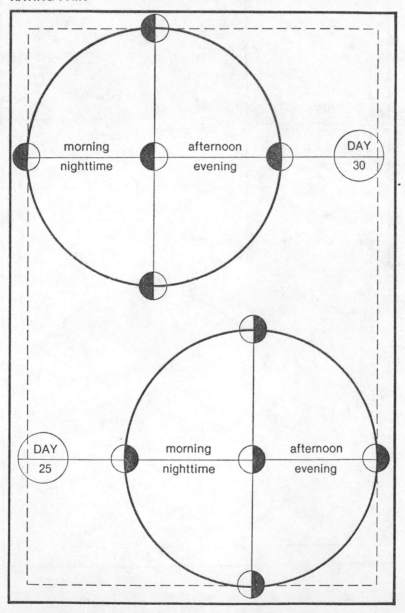

RATING PAIN

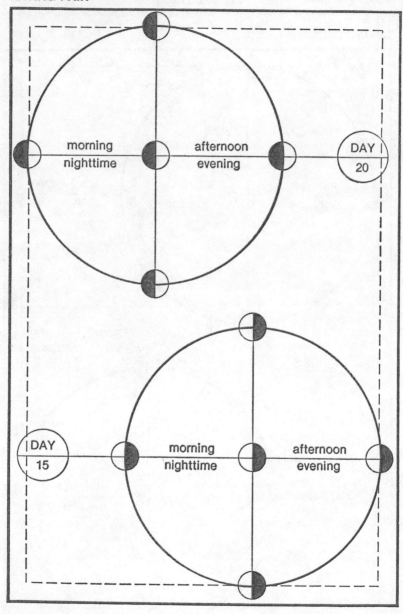

RATING PAIN

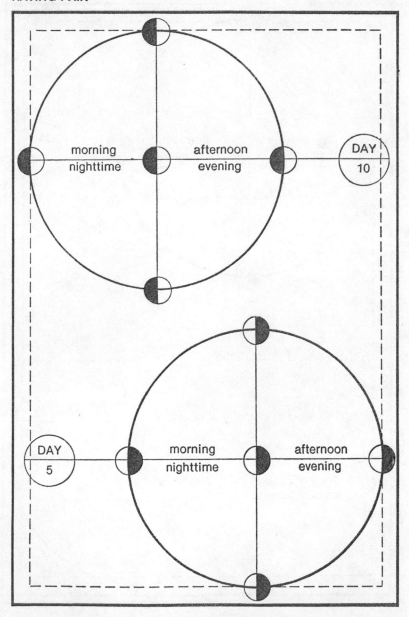

RATING PAIN

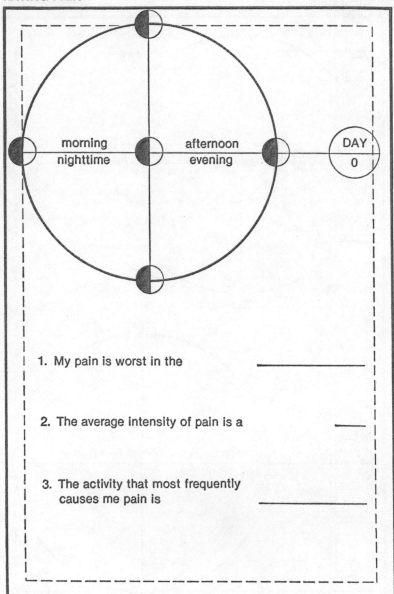

1. My pain is worst in the _____

2. The average intensity of pain is a _____

3. The activity that most frequently
   causes me pain is _____

ACTIVITY RECORD — DAY 30

WHEN	WHAT	WHERE	WITH WHOM	PAIN BETTER	PAIN WORSE
First awakening					
Mid-morning					
Noon					
Afternoon					
Evening					
Nighttime					

ACTIVITY RECORD

DAY 25

WHEN	WHAT	WHERE	WITH WHOM	PAIN BETTER	PAIN WORSE
First awakening					
Mid-morning					
Noon					
Afternoon					
Evening					
Nighttime					

ACTIVITY RECORD

DAY 20

WHEN	WHAT	WHERE	WITH WHOM	PAIN BETTER	PAIN WORSE
First awakening					
Mid-morning					
Noon					
Afternoon					
Evening					
Nighttime					

ACTIVITY RECORD DAY 15

WHEN	WHAT	WHERE	WITH WHOM	PAIN BETTER	PAIN WORSE
First awakening					
Mid-morning					
Noon					
Afternoon					
Evening					
Nighttime					

ACTIVITY RECORD						
WHEN	WHAT	WHERE	WITH WHOM	PAIN BETTER	PAIN WORSE	DAY 10
First awakening						
Mid-morning						
Noon						
Afternoon						
Evening						
Nighttime						

ACTIVITY RECORD

DAY 5

WHEN	WHAT	WHERE	WITH WHOM	PAIN BETTER	PAIN WORSE
First awakening					
Mid-morning					
Noon					
Afternoon					
Evening					
Nighttime					

ACTIVITY RECORD

DAY 0

WHEN	WHAT	WHERE	WITH WHOM	PAIN BETTER	PAIN WORSE
First awakening					
Mid-morning					
Noon					
Afternoon					
Evening					
Nighttime					

PAIN TOLERANCE TABLE		
Activities	Hours/Day	Pain Rating
Walking		
Sexual Activity		
Light Housework		
Cooking/Meal Preparation		
Mild Exercise (Physical Therapy)		
Gardening/House Repairs		
Marketing/Errands		
Entertaining		
Handling Job Responsibilities		
Playing with Children		

The three most painful Pain Enhancers are:

1

2

3

PAIN TOLERANCE TABLE		
Passivities	Hours/Day	Pain Rating
Sleeping		
Lying in Bed Awake		
Sitting/Reading		
Sitting/Idle		
Sitting/Car		
Watching T.V.		
Napping		
On Telephone		
Pacing Floor		
Lying on Couch		

The three most relaxing Pain Reducers are:

1

2

3

Name of Medicine	Reason for Use	Drug Effect Positive	Drug Effect Negative
1			
2			
3			
4			
5			
6			

Name of Medicine	Reason for Use	Drug Effect Positive	Drug Effect Negative
7			
8			
9			
10			
11			
12			

Name of Medicine	Day 1				Day 2				Day 3				Day 4				Day 5				Day 6				Day 7			
	M	A	E	N	M	A	E	N	M	A	E	N	M	A	E	N	M	A	E	N	M	A	E	N	M	A	E	N

RELAXATION RATING

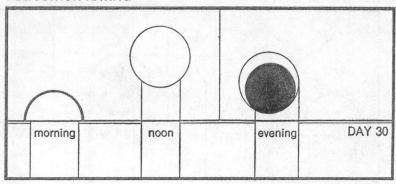

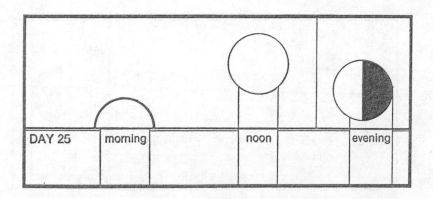

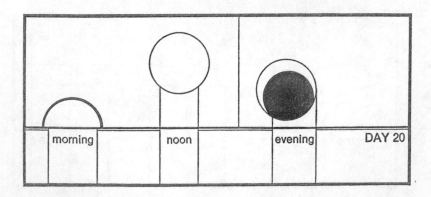

RELAXATION RATING

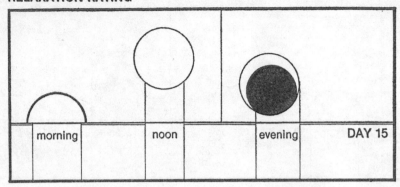

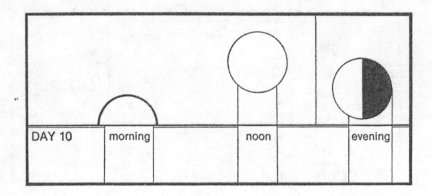

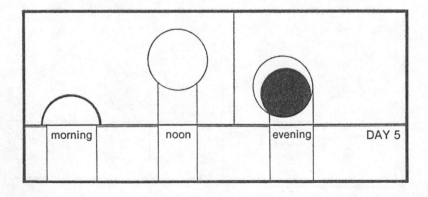

RELAXATION RATING

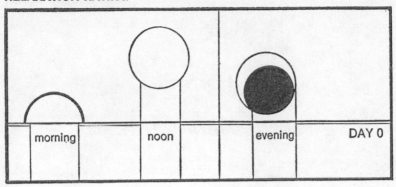

| morning | noon | evening | DAY 0 |

1. The time of day I am best able to relax Is _____

2. My average level of relaxation is a   _____

3. The activity that most frequently
   helps me to relax is   _____

Appendix B

USEFUL MEDICAL TERMS

The following glossary defines and amplifies those newer treatments mentioned throughout the book. It is provided to help you keep abreast of the latest medical advances and to help you understand the components of the new pain treatments. It is divided into four sections: diagnostic tests, surgical terms, physical therapies, and behavioral therapies.

DIAGNOSTIC TESTS

CAT SCAN The computerized axial tomogram is a new technique for visualizing the soft tissues of the body—the muscles, tendons, and organs, as opposed to the harder bone. Ordinary X rays can "see" bones well because they are of a much higher density than the softer structures around them. The organs of the body thus come out relatively gray or black on a regular X ray while the bone shows up white. An X ray is really a negative; the X rays are stopped by the bone and the areas where they do not hit show up as white. The CAT scanner enables us to see cross sections of the body just as if we sliced a grapefruit in half and looked at its cross section. The organs, bones, and ligaments show up as if we were looking at an anatomy book. This is accomplished by having the X-ray machine take many X rays through the same plane from different points. This information is then fed to the computer, which "enhances" or magnifies details many times to produce the clarity of the final X ray. The CAT scanner's greatest use is in areas that in the past had to be diagnosed by surgery or biopsy. We can now see the organs that in X rays look gray and blended with the surrounding tissue, with almost the same detail and clarity as a picture. The coned-down CAT scanner is a scanner with a special attachment that allows us to see the smaller areas of the spinal canal and its surrounding structures with greater clarity and magnification. This newer technique, when fully refined, may enable us to see a herniated disk without the use of a myelogram. The disadvantages of a CAT scanner are that it is expensive and that at times it cannot show us the fine details we need to see.

DISKOGRAM A newer technique that involves injection of contrast material into the disk itself to outline its structures and to check for physical integrity. It, too, is not foolproof, and it has the side effects of producing its own structural damage to the disk. It has, however, become a valuable research tool and may become a more useful medical tool in the future.

ELECTROMYOGRAM (EMG) Gives us an indication of how well a nerve is functioning and, conversely how much damage has been done to that nerve. Nerve impulses pass along a nerve electrochemically, that is, through chemical storage and transmission of electricity. These impulses can be picked up on the oscilloscope. We know what normal patterns look like, and we can match a person's curve to normal and abnormal curves to discover how much damage has occurred and how much recovery can be expected. It is useful in looking for damaged or herniated disks.

MYELOGRAM An X ray of the spine. Metallic contrast solution is injected into the spinal canal and around the spinal cord, giving shape and definition to the cord's structures. Using this method, any protrusion of a herniated disk becomes visible as a bulge and a column of contrast material. It is not foolproof, but it does offer us a fairly reliable tool for visualizing physical problems in the spinal canal.

THERMOGRAM An X-ray tool used to look at the different temperatures of the body. The temperatures of different areas of the body differ because of greater or diminished blood supply to that area. For instance, an area of the finger that has been damaged will show up as having more blood supply since the body attempted to heal the injury. On a thermogram, injury shows a different-colored area from the surrounding tissue, indicating that the body's restorative powers are being concentrated in that area. It is also used in detecting areas that are difficult to examine directly.

VENOGRAM   Contrast material is injected into the rich plexus, or network of veins, surrounding the spinal cord. Any defect shows up as a space-distorting mass that make the veins deviate from their normal course.

A SHORT AND PAINLESS COMPENDIUM OF
SURGICAL TERMS

Surgical procedures are needed, useful, and curative at times. Surgeons by and large respect the fact that pain may recur after surgery. The surgical terms you should be familiar with and able to use in asking your doctor questions are set forth below. Remember to ask. Be an informed consumer of medicine and surgery.

CORDOTOMY AND RHIZOTOMY   Procedures used to cut a nerve or nerve tract in the spinal cord. They are used late in the course of chronic pain and usually the pain recurs after they have been done. These procedures have not been shown to be effective. Approach them with caution.

FUSION   Often done in conjunction with a laminectomy. Fusion is used when excessive bone is removed and the spine is deemed to be unstable. Then, a bridge of bone taken from your wing bone or ilium is placed across two vertebrae in such a way that the graft and the two vertebrae fuse, thereby giving added structure and support to the spinal column that has been stressed beyond stability.

HERNIATED DISK   This is also known as a "ruptured" or "slipped" disk. In reality, the disk is like a golf ball filled with gelatin, only much flatter. With age or trauma or from unknown causes, the outer ring of the disk, which is hard, begins to fragment, and the jelly inside leaks out. The jelly then may impinge on a nerve or surrounding structures, causing pain. It is this outer ring that "ruptures." *Most back pain is not caused by disk problems.* Most back pain can be treated well without surgery.

LAMINECTOMY   This is an operation on the spine, most often done to remove pieces of a herniated disk. Laminectomy refers to the removal of the lamina—a piece of the vertebra, or backbone —to expose the nerve and disk underneath. Laminectomies are most often performed after a myelogram has revealed a herniated disk. Sometimes they are performed with very little evidence of a surgical problem. Repeated laminectomies, as a rule, are to be avoided as scarring, called arachnoiditis, occurs frequently, and pain can be worse after the surgery than before. It is often to your advantage to get a second opinion. No surgeon who is truly concerned with your welfare will mind this measure of extra care.

PERCUTANEOUS DISKECTOMY This is a relatively new technique, using microsurgery to remove the debris of a herniated disk through a minute opening instead of through a large surgical scar. It is a new procedure, and its results are just being evaluated at the present time.

PHYSICAL THERAPIES

Two of the newest physical treatments, nerve block and transcutaneous nerve stimulation—in combination with each other and alone—have given us valuable new tools in the fight against chronic pain.

SPINAL BLOCK A preparation of cortisone and novocaine is injected directly into the spinal canal. Novocaine will deaden pain and cortisone will decrease inflammation surrounding the diseased nerve roots. The needle is inserted below the level of the end of the spinal cord but before the sac covering the cord's ends (anatomically, this occurs about four inches up from the base of the tailbone, or coccyx). The novocaine used is similar to that injected when a tooth is filled, but it is in a different form, called procaine. A differential spinal block is also a diagnostic tool. Using different amounts of procaine, a physician can determine from where along the pain pathway the pain signals are emanating. Every fifteen minutes a different strength is used. We know from experience that when a patient reports relief at a certain strength, the pain is due to the nerve portion of the pain system. If it is relieved at another strength, then the pain is produced along more central pathways that intersect with these nerve pathways. At still another strength, it would indicate that the pain is produced by a chain of sympathetic nerves which produce burning pain down the leg. A series of these blocks, or just one or two, may alleviate the pain for up to six months and allow other parts of the treatment to progress. They constitute a promising tool.

TRANSCUTANEOUS NERVE STIMULATION (TNS) A recent treatment that makes use of the gate theory (see Section 2). The TNS unit consists of a small box about the size of a cigarette pack that is worn on the belt. Wires from the box lead to plastic disks taped to the skin, through which a mild electric current passes when the patient turns the dial. This current overrides pain impulses that are triggered along the nerve pathways and blocks them at the spinal gate. The gate closes to all impulses coming along the nerve pathways leading to it when it is overloaded; the electric current, which is felt as a mild tingling or buzzing, overloads the circuit and closes the gate. The patient can wear the machine all day, but may turn it on only for a few hours. The amount of time may be limited by irritation, which tends to form around the disks in some patients.

Let us go back to our automobile analogy. If at a tollgate six Chevrolets jam the entrance and the tollgate closes, then not only the six Chevrolets (the electric current) but all of the Chryslers, Cadillacs, and Toyotas (pain, heat) cannot get through either. TNS works for about 50 to 60 percent of those who try it. It is a safe, effective, and nonsurgical way to reduce pain without medication.

BEHAVIORAL THERAPIES

The most recent and perhaps the most promising of the new treatments lie in the area of behavioral therapy. Combined with the physical approaches, these new behavioral methods are reshaping treatment. Your awareness of them will help you to become a better pain-treatment consumer.

BIOFEEDBACK A teaching method using the latest technology. It "feeds back" to the patient, through sound, light, or a needle on a scale, information about muscles, skin temperatures, or brain waves. This information is usually involuntary and unavailable to the patient. The biofeedback machine is able to graphically demonstrate to the patient changes in his or her involuntary functions, such as muscle tone, skin temperature, or brain waves. Through training with a technician, the patient then learns to control these biological functions and thereby control the functions themselves. The patient learns to control muscle tension, skin temperature, even blood pressure. Think of the implications! You can learn to control functions which were once thought to be strictly involuntary. For instance, if you were asked to relax your forehead muscle, there would be considerable effort and you probably would fail. If you were asked to change the temperature of your skin now and make it ten degrees colder, you would probably look strangely at the person who asked you to do so and then walk away. Yet patients trained in biofeedback can do just that. It is a well-proven although new technique—a legitimate tool in pain reduction. This is a useful tool in migraine patients, particularly as it relates to controlling skin temperature. Migraine headaches are dependent to a large extent on the dilation of the small vessels of the brain. Learning to control this physiological function helps control both skin temperature and migraine because of the underlying problem, which is an instability in opening and closing of the arterioles.

The principles behind biofeedback are the same as those used in learning theory: immediate knowledge of success or failure in trying to lower skin temperature or muscle spasm teaches what is successful and what is not, and increases the likelihood of repeating successful behavior. In addition to this theoretical underpinning, biofeedback also uses repetitive successful trials to reinforce involuntary physiological functions. These functions would never have been able to be monitored if they were not first, however, turned into the intermediate stimulus of sound or light.

BEHAVIOR MODIFICATION When you decide to change your eating habits so that you cut out a midafternoon snack and you do it by altering your time schedule so that you eat lunch a little later than usual to cut down the hunger, you are using behavior modification. When you wean a baby off a bottle by slowly substituting other oral gratifications and giving him a cup instead, you are modifying behavior. Behavior modification combines sound psychological principles with common sense with the intention of changing behavior. It has nothing to do with the forced conditioning of Pavlov or the Freudian analysis that is caricatured so often. There are, for instance, several behavior-modification diets. Below are two examples:

It has been found that overweight persons tend to eat quickly and do not give themselves a chance to feel satisfied. A modification in this behavior would be to stop a meal at midpoint and push the food away for five minutes. If, at the end of that time, you feel satisfied, then leave the rest on the dish. If you are still hungry, continue the meal.

It has also been found that overweight persons are often "field-dependent." That is, they take their hunger cues from the environment rather than from internal sources. These persons have difficulty in gauging weight changes of less than five to eight pounds—very damaging for anyone wanting to diet. A behavior solution: buy a scale and use it every day to give you the cues you would not find internally.

These two examples give some idea of how behavioral modification might work. There are behavioral paths that apply to chronic pain sufferers as well. They include treating pain behaviors as *habits* which can be broken without undue strain on your willpower. They are designed to be used at home or at work, and you do not need special equipment or experts to help you. For instance:

1. Make a list of five pain behaviors. These are behaviors that you exhibit because you are in pain and would not otherwise show. For instance, staying in bed half the morning or having your spouse make a telephone call you would ordinarily make, or avoiding going out occasionally. Change one behavior a week for the next five weeks but keep working on the previous week's behavior so that by the end of five weeks you have changed five behaviors. You will be surprised at how your perception of pain changes and how others' perception of you changes.

Bill Herbert was a salesman for a large communications company. One of his pain behaviors was to constantly pull and grab at his left arm to indicate that he was in pain. Without analyzing why he did this, he was urged to stop the pain behavior. He did, and within four days, three of his coworkers indicated to him that "somehow you look better." He began to feel more accepted and productive.

2. Pick one habit that you want to change—smoking, overeating, or watching television too many hours a day—and modify it in a special way. Change your brand of cigarettes, or modify your eating habits as we discussed. Change one behavioral bit (remember, small, manageable bits) at a time and pick another in sequence the following week, until you arrive at your goal. Make a list of the way or sequence in which you want to arrive at that goal. Make it a reachable one. It will give you a sense of mastery of your own body, and with it a sense that you can change your pain habits.

3. Stop using the word pain for one week. You may find that you do not need to use it as much in the future.

4. Start doing one task you gave up to another family member because of pain. Start with something small.

5. The next time you start to ask for a favor because of your pain, *don't*.

The five examples above are simple and straightforward and may seem easy. *They are not.* They take dedication and motivation. But, once begun, you will be better able to manage your pain. Used in conjunction with other therapies, behavior modification can be of great help in decreasing chronic pain.

EMOTIONAL THERAPIES

When people hear the word psychological, they often think of classical Freudian analysis—on the couch for five to seven years. Without a doubt, this kind of analysis has nothing to offer the chronic pain sufferer.

The newer methods of treatment in the emotional realm involve the use of brief-term therapies designed to help the patient formulate goals, or change attitudes about behavior. Special group therapies with a goal-oriented thrust have been devised for the chronic pain sufferer. These group therapies also offer pain patients the chance to end their feelings of isolation by speaking with other chronic victims. Dr. Peter Sifneos, a noted Harvard psychiatrist, has devised several brief-term therapies. They are time-limited, usually eight to twelve weeks, and address one or two issues. The therapist helps the patient to define goals, or areas he would like to change, and the twelve weeks are devoted to achieving those goals, or at least finding the right track. It is an ideal therapy for the pain sufferer for several reasons. First, Dr. Sifneos discovered that some patients are not able to express their feelings in words, but instead express them in terms of bodily symptoms. Many patients with chronic pain suffer from this handicap and the brief-term type of therapy is ideally suited to helping them to begin to turn symptoms into feelings.

Pat, a forty-three-year-old housewife and a chronic pain sufferer, began experiencing increasing amounts of back pain when her son left the house for college. Clearly, Pat had back pain, diagnosed years before as a residue from a herniated disk. Just as clearly, however, Pat was depressed about her son finally growing up and leaving home. Her family recognized this but Pat was constitutionally unable to express feelings in words; she expressed it in terms of something with which she was familiar —pain.

Pat entered a course of brief-term therapy and was able to begin to verbalize some of the sadness and loneliness she felt. As she did this, her pain became less of a focal point and she was able to resume her role as wife and mother.

Two other forms of psychological therapy are available now to the chronic pain sufferer. Group therapy is one, but a special kind of group therapy. Groups are composed of from eight to fourteen persons and are a combination of education, behavior modification, and shared experiences. Family members are often invited to come and share their experiences. Behavioral tests are given, almost as homework, and patients are expected to change and work hard at changing. These groups can be exciting, dynamic forums where patients can openly share with one another their pain experiences and decrease their sense of isolation and loneliness. In our experience, 60 percent of the people involved in these groups are able to make some changes in their life-styles as a result of such an experience. The change may be a small one—such as making dinner two evenings a week more than before—or a major one—such as returning to work. The universal feeling, however, among persons enrolled in such groups, is that they are able to come out with a new understanding and an increased ability to manage pain.

FAMILY THERAPY

Pain sufferers do not live in a vacuum. They live with other people, usually family. A family is a unit, another type of system, and it too feels the hurt of chronic pain and the soothing of relief. As we learned before, the family can be beneficial or it can be detrimental when it comes to controlling pain. In either case, it is part and parcel of the pain system. Any attempt to treat pain without treating the family is like treating bronchitis without taking into account the air quality. The environment *must* be taken into account. We find that the patient is usually surprised at the family's willingness to participate in therapy. Comments such as "I can't impose on them anymore" and "I don't think they're interested" are often contradicted by the family's eagerness to engage in therapy with the patient.

BIBLIOGRAPHY

ARNOFF, G., and WILSON, R. "How to Teach Your Patients to Control Chronic Pain," *Behavioral Medicine,* July 1978, pp. 29–35.

BATESON, G. *Mind and Nature.* New York: E. P. Dutton, 1979.

BLOCK, A. "Behavioral Treatment of Chronic Pain: Variables Affecting Treatment and Efficacy," *Pain* 8 (1980):367–75.

BURCHFIELD, S. "The Stress Response: A New Perspective," *Psychosomatic Medicine* 41 (Dec. 1979):661–71.

COELHO, G.; HAMBURG, D., and ADAMS, J. *Coping and Adaptation.* New York: Basic Books, 1974.

COUSINS, N. *Anatomy of an Illness As Perceived by the Patient.* New York: W. W. Norton, 1979.

DELESON-JONES, F., and MAAS, J. "Diagnostic Subgroups of Affective Disorders," *American Journal of Psychiatry* 132 (Nov. 1975):11.

ENGLE, G. "Psychogenic Pain in the Pain Prone Patient," *American Journal of Medicine* 26 (1959):898.

GESSELY, A. "Tension Control for Pain," *Psychosomatics* 21 (Nov. 1980):11.

GOODMAN, L., and GILLMAN, A. *The Pharmacologic Basis of Therapeutics.* 6th ed. New York: Macmillan, 1980.

GRACELY, R. H. "Psychophysiological Assessment of Human Pain." In *Advances in Pain Research and Therapy,* edited by Bonica, J. J.; Liebeskind, J. C., and Albe-Fessard, D., 3:805–24. New York: Raven Press, 1979.

———. "Pain Measurement in Man." In *Pain Discomfort and Humanitarian Care,* edited by Ng, L., and Bonica, J. J. New York: Elsevier/Excerpta Medica/North-Holland, 1980.

GRACELY, R. H.; DUBNER, R.; MCGRATH, P., and HEFT, M. "New Methods of Pain Measurements and Their Application to Pain Control," *International Dental Journal* 28 (1978):52–65.

GRACELY, R. H.; MCGRATH, P., and DUBNER, R. "Ratio Skills with Sensory and Affective Verbal Pain Descriptors," *Pain* 5 (1978):5–18.

———. "Narcotic Analgesia: Fentanyl: Reduces the Intensity but Not the Unpleasantness of Painful Twofold Sensations," *Science* 203 (1979):1261–63.

HACKETT, P. "The Surgeon and the Difficult Pain Problem," *International Psychiatric Clinics* 4 (1967):179–88.

HENDREN, R. KRUPP. "Psychiatry and Pain Management Programs," *Psychosomatics* 20 (Apr. 1979):229–32.

HIGHLAND, E. "Neodissection Interpretation of Pain Reaction and Hypnosis," *Psychological Review* 80 (1973):396–441.

HILL, D., ed. *Physiology, Emotion and Psychosomatic Illness.* CIBA Symposium. New York: Elsevier/Excerpta Medica/North-Holland, 1972.

HOLMES, T. H., and RAHE, R. "The Life Adjustment Rating Scale," *Journal of Psychosomatic Research* 11 (1967):213–18.

HOUDE, R. "Non-Narcotic Terms for Controlling Pain," *Progress in Cancer Treatment in Drug Therapy,* Aug. 1980, p. 59.

JANIS, I. *Psychological Stress.* New York: John Wiley and Sons, 1958.

KINSTON, M. "Bodily Communication and Psychotherapy: A Psychosomatic Approach," *International Journal of Psychiatry and Medicine* 6 (1975):195–201.

MACDONALD, A. "Abnormally Tender Muscle Regions and Associated Painful Movements," *Pain* 8 (1980):197–205.

MARUTA, T., and OSBORNE, D. "Sexual Activity and Chronic Pain Patients," *Psychosomatics* 19 (Sept. 1978):531.

MASON, D., and GUTHRIE, H., eds. "The Medicine Called Nutrition," *Symposium of Medev Medical Education Program.* Westport, Conn.: Medical Education Programs, 1979.

The Medical Letter on Drugs and Therapeutics 23 (Jan. 1981): Issue 574.

MELZAK, R. *The Puzzle of Pain.* New York: Basic Books, 1973.

MELZAK, R., and WALL, P. D. "Pain Mechanics: A New Theory," *Science* 150 (1965):971–79.

MERSKY, H. "Psychological Aspects of Pain," *Post Graduate Medical Journal* 44 (1968):297–306.

Moos, R. *Coping with Physical Illness*. New York: Plenum Medical Book Company, 1977.

Murphy, L., and Moriarty, A. *Vulnerability, Coping, and Growth: From Infancy to Adolescence*. New Haven: Yale University Press, 1976.

Nigl, A., and Fischer-Williams, M. "The Treatment of Low Back Strain with Electromyographic Biofeedback in Relaxation Training," *Psychosomatics* 21 (June 1980):495.

Painter, J.; Seres, J., and Newman, R. "Assessing Benefits of the Pain Center: Why Some Patients Regress," *Pain* 8 (1980): 108–13.

Pinsky, J. "Behavioral Consequences of Chronic Intractable Benign Pain," *Behavioral Medicine* 7 (May 1980):12–18.

Rees, L. "Stress, Distress, and Disease," *The British Journal of Psychiatry* 128 (1976):3–18.

Roberts, A., and Rainhardt, L. "The Behavioral Management of Chronic Pain: And Long Term Followup with Comparison Groups," *Pain* 8 (1962):151–62.

Seres, J., and Newman, R. "The Results of Treatment of Chronic Low Back Pain at Portland Pain Center," *Journal of Neurosurgery* 45 (July 1976):33–36.

Simmons, R. "Pain Medication Contracts for Problem Patients," *Psychosomatics* 20 (Feb. 1979):122–30.

Smoller, B., and Schulman, B. "Chronic Pain: Prevention Through Early Intervention," *Occupational Health and Safety* 50 (Mar. 1981):14–22.

Snyder, S. "Opiate and Benzodiazepine Receptors," *Psychosomatics* 22 (Nov. 1981):986–93.

Specht, E. "Conservative Management of Low Back Pain," *Southern Medical Journal* 69 (Mar. 1976):334–36.

Sternbach, R. *Pain Patients (Traits and Treatments)*. New York: Academic Press, 1974.

Sternbach, R., and Pinsky, J. "More About the Chronic Pain Patient," *Journal of Human Stress* 4 (Sept. 1978).

Swanson, D.; Swenson, W.; Maruta, T., and McPhee, M. "Program for Managing Chronic Pain, Program Description and Characteristics of Patients at the Mayo Clinic," *Mayo Clinic Proceedings* 51 (July 1976):401–11.

Swanson, D., and Maruta, T. "Patients Complaining of Extreme Pain," *Mayo Clinic Proceedings* 55 (Feb. 1980):563–66.

SWEET, W. H. "Some Current Problems in Pain Research and Therapy," *Pain* 10 (June 1981):297–309.

TAHMOUSH, A. J. "Causalgia: A Redefinition of a Clinical Pain Syndrome," *Pain* 10 (Apr. 1980): 187–97.

VAILLANT, G. *Adaptation to Life*. Boston: Little, Brown, 1977.

WEISENBERG, M. *Pain: Clinical and Experimental Perspectives*. St. Louis: C. V. Mosby Company, 1975.

INDEX

["